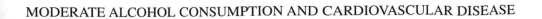

MODERATE ALCOHOL CONSUMPTION AND CARDIOVASCULAR DISEASE

# Medical Science Symposia Series

Volume 15

# Moderate Alcohol Consumption and Cardiovascular Disease

*Edited by*

R. Paoletti
*Institute of Pharmacological Sciences, University of Milan, Milan, Italy*

A.L. Klatsky
*Kaiser Permanente Medical Center, Oakland, California, U.S.A.*

A. Poli
*Nutrition Foundation of Italy, Milan, Italy*

and

S. Zakhari
*National Institute of Alcohol Abuse and Alcoholism,
National Institutes of Health, Bethesda, Maryland, U.S.A.*

KLUWER ACADEMIC PUBLISHERS
DORDRECHT / BOSTON / LONDON

Fondazione Giovanni Lorenzini, Medical Science Foundation, Milan, Italy
Giovanni Lorenzini Medical Foundation, Houston, Texas, U.S.A.

*CENTRO STUDI DELL'ALIMENTAZIONE*
*NUTRITION FOUNDATION OF ITALY*

A C.I.P. Catalogue record for this book is available from the Library of Congress.

ISBN 0-7923-6572-0

Published by Kluwer Academic Publishers,
P.O. Box 17, 3300 AA Dordrecht, The Netherlands.

Sold and distributed in North, Central and South America
by Kluwer Academic Publishers,
101 Philip Drive, Norwell, MA 02061, U.S.A.

In all other countries, sold and distributed
by Kluwer Academic Publishers,
P.O. Box 322, 3300 AH Dordrecht, The Netherlands.

*Printed on acid-free paper*

Printed in the Netherlands.

CONTENTS

The effects of alcohol consumption on human health have fuelled a vigorous scientific debate in recent years. This volume, based on the scientific sessions of the International Meeting on MODERATE ALCOHOL CONSUMPTION AND CARDIOVASCULAR DISEASE, held in Venice October 30-31, 1999, is intended to offer an up-to-date view of the most recent information on this complex topic.

While comprehension of the damages associated with alcohol abuse has improved, an increasing number of epidemiological studies performed in different countries of the world, have shown that individuals consuming moderate amounts of alcohol (10-30 g/day, approximately equivalent to not more than two drinks per day in men and one drink per day in women) are less affected by acute coronary events than total abstainers. The apparent protection is evident (the rate of coronary events in most studies is reduced by about 30%) and has been observed and documented among various population groups (men, women, several racial groups, middle-aged and older individuals). Protection is seen in patients with no known history of coronary heart disease, as well as in those with coronary heart disease, diabetes, etc. Recent data suggest that the protection induced by a moderate alcohol use extends to the risk of ischemic strokes and of ischemic damage to the lower limbs. Since adverse alcohol effects are less frequent at these low daily intakes, total mortality is also favourably affected in moderate alcohol consumers as compared to abstainers.

The mechanisms underlying the antiatherogenic effects of alcohol are now better understood. Alcohol consumption significantly and consistently raises the plasma levels of the antiatherogenic HDL lipoproteins. The tendency to thrombosis is also favourably affected (partially via decreased plasma fibrinogen levels), while the efficiency of fibrinolytic pathways seems to be improved.

An ongoing debate focuses on the possible additional antiatherosclerotic effects of some nonalcohol component of specific alcoholic beverages. The antioxidant effects of a few minor components of wine (and especially red wine) may contribute to the antiatherosclerotic action of this beverage, modulating the processes leading to LDL oxidation and eventually to the formation, growth, and maturation of the atherosclerotic plaque. The role of beverage choice remains unresolved.

We hope this volume of *Proceeding* from the International Meeting on MODERATE ALCOHOL CONSUMPTION AND CARDIOVASCULAR DISEASE will be of help to the clinicians and researchers interested in this fascinating area of human behaviour.

The editors would like to thank Ann Jackson of the GIOVANNI LORENZINI MEDICAL FOUNDATION for her editorial coordination and assistance in the preparation of this volume.

*The Editors*

LIST OF CONTRIBUTORS

Christie M. Ballantyne, *Department of Medicine, Baylor College of Medicine, MS A-601, 6565 Fannin Street, Houston, Texas 77030, USA*

Diane H. Bick, *Department of Medicine, Baylor College of Medicine, MS A-601, 6565 Fannin Street, Houston, Texas 77030, USA*

François Cambien, *Sc 7 INSERM, 17 rue du Fer à Moulin, 75005 Paris, France*

Michael H. Criqui, M.D., M.P.H., *UCSD School of Medicine, 9500 Gilman Drive, Dept #0607, La Jolla, California 92093, USA*

Patrick Duriez, *Département de Recherches sur les Lipoprotéines et l'Athérosclérose, INSERM U325, Institut Pasteur, 1 rue du Professeur Calmette, BP 245, 59019 Lille, France*

Christian Ehnholm, *National Public Health Institute, Department of Biochemistry, Mannerheimintie 166, FIN-00300 Helsinki, Finland*

Jean-Charles Fruchart, *Département de Recherches sur les Lipoprotéines et l'Athérosclérose, INSERM U325, Institut Pasteur, 1 rue du Professeur Calmette, BP 245, 59019 Lille, France*

Morten Grønbæk, M.D., Ph.D., *Copenhagen Centre for Prospective Population Studies, Danish Epidemiology Science Centre at the Institute of Preventive Medicine, Copenhagen University Hospital, H:S Kommunehospitalet, Copenhagen, Denmark*

Jane Henley M.S.P.H., *Department of Epidemiology and Surveillance Research, American Cancer Society, 1599 Clifton Road, NE, Atlanta, Georgia 30329, USA*

Hiroshige Itakura, *National Institute of Health and Nutrition, 2-6-36 Hayamiya, Nerima-ku, Tokyo 179-0085, Japan*

Matti Jauhiainen, *National Public Health Institute, Department of Biochemistry, Mannerheimintie 166, FIN-00300 Helsinki, Finland*

Kay T. Kimball, *Department of Medicine, Baylor College of Medicine, MS A-601, 6565 Fannin Street, Houston, Texas 77030, USA*

Arthur L. Klatsky, M.D., *Kaiser Permanente Medical Center, 280 West MacArthur Boulevard, Oakland, California 94611, USA*

Cornelis Kluft, *Gaubius Laboratory, TNO-PG, P.O. Box 2215, 2301 CE Leiden, The Netherlands*

Kazuo Kondo, *National Institute of Health and Nutrition, Tokyo, Japan*

Markku Kupari, M.D., *Division of Cardiology, Department of Medicine, Helsinki University Central*

*Hospital, 00290 Helsinki, Finland*

Akiyo Matsumoto, *National Institute of Health and Nutrition, Tokyo, Japan*

Emma A. Meagher, M.D., *Center for Experimental Therapeutics, 9053 Gates Building, 3400 Spruce Street, Philadelphia, Pennsylvania 19140, USA.*

Kari Poikolainen, *Järvenpää Addiction Hospital, 04480 Haarajoki, Finland*

Henry J. Pownall, Ph.D., *Section of Atherosclerosis and Lipoprotein Research, Department of Medicine, Baylor College of Medicine, MS A-601, 6565 Fannin Street, Houston, Texas 77030, USA*

Gerald M. Reaven, M.D., *213 East Grand Avenue, South San Francisco, California 94080, USA*

Eric Rimm, Sc.D., *Departments of Epidemiology and Nutrition, Harvard School of Public Health, 665 Huntington Avenue, Boston, Massachusetts 02115, USA*

Aron Rosenthal, *Department of Epidemiology and Surveillance Research,          American Cancer Society, 1599 Clifton Road, NE, Atlanta, Georgia 30329, USA*

A. Gerald Shaper, *Royal Free and University College Medical School, London NW3 2PF, UK*

Meir J. Stampfer, M.D., Dr.P.H., *Departments of Epidemiology and Nutrition, Harvard School of Public Health and Channing Laboratory, Department of Medicine, Brigham and Women's Hospital and Harvard Medical School, 181 Longwood Avenue, Boston, Massachusetts 02115, USA*

Michael J. Thun, M.D., M.S., *Department of Epidemiology and Surveillance Research, American Cancer Society, 1599 Clifton Road, NE, Atlanta, Georgia 30329, USA*

S. Goya Wannamethee, *Royal Free and University College Medical School, London NW3 2PF, UK*

Danièle Zoch, *Section of Atherosclerosis and Lipoprotein Research, Department of Medicine, Baylor College of Medicine, MS A-601, 6565 Fannin Street, Houston, Texas 77030, USA*

# Alcohol and Cardiovascular Diseases: An Historical Overview

Arthur L. Klatsky

## Introduction

Always intrinsically interesting, study of the history of a subject also seldom fails to provide insights about current knowledge. Perhaps the most important result is realization of past mistakes, with the potential for avoiding their repetition. Past attempts to generalize and simplify the subject of alcohol and cardiovascular diseases have, in several areas, slowed progress in understanding this area. Disparity in relations of alcohol drinking to various cardiovascular conditions [1] has become increasingly clear. Underlying all alcohol-health relationships is the basic disparity between the effects of lighter and heavier drinking. In this selective background historical overview, the following will be considered separately: cardiomyopathy, arsenic and cobalt beer drinkers' disease, cardiovascular beri-beri, systemic hypertension, cardiac arrhythmias, cerebrovascular disease, atherosclerotic coronary heart disease (CHD), total mortality, and definitions of safe drinking limits.

## Alcoholic Cardiomyopathy

An apparent relationship between chronic intake of large amounts of alcohol and heart disease was noted by several distinguished 19th century physicians [2-6]. Of special note is the term "Munchener bierherz,, coined by the German pathologist Bollinger [7]. Bollinger described cardiac dilatation and hypertrophy among Bavarian beer drinkers, who consumed an average of 432 liters of beer per year, compared to 82 liters in per year other parts of Germany.

Graham Steell [5] in a report of 25 cases, stated "not only do I recognize alcoholism as one of the causes of muscle failure of the heart but I find it a comparatively common one." Several years later, in 1900, an epidemic of heart disease due to arsenic contaminated beer occurred in Manchester, England. Following the arsenic-beer episode Steell [8] wrote "in the production of the combined affection of the peripheral nerves and the heart met with in beer drinkers, arsenic has been shown to play a conspicuous part." In another textbook, *The Study of the Pulse*, the great William MacKenzie [9] described cases of heart failure attributed to alcohol and first used the term "alcoholic heart disease." Although there was general doubt that alcohol had a direct role in producing heart muscle disease early in the twentieth century, some [10] took a strong view in favor of such a relationship.

1

R. Paoletti et al. (eds.), Moderate Alcohol Consumption and Cardiovascular Disease, 1–9.

The concept of "beri-beri heart disease" dominated thinking about alcohol and the heart for several decades after descriptions of cardiovascular beri-beri [11-12]. For the past 50 years increasing interest has been evident in possible direct toxicity of alcohol upon the myocardial cells, independent of, or, in addition to, deficiency states. The sheer volume of clinical observations, plus evidence of decreased myocardial function in heavy chronic drinkers, and a few good controlled studies have now solidly established the concept of alcoholic cardiomyopathy. Since the entity is indistinguishable from other forms of dilated cardiomyopathy, the absence of diagnostic tests remains a major impediment to epidemiologic study. Most cases of dilated cardiomyopathy in 1999 are of unknown cause, with a postviral autoimmune process and a genetic predisposition the leading etiologic hypotheses. There is convincing circumstantial evidence of nonspecific cardiac abnormalities related to alcohol in animals and humans. The landmark study of Urbano-Marquez et al. [13] showed a clear relation of lifetime alcohol consumption to structural and functional myocardial and skeletal muscle abnormalities in alcoholics. The amounts of alcohol needed were large—the equivalent of 120 grams alcohol/day for 20 years. Thus, Walsche's term "cirrhosis of the heart" [3] seems very appropriate.

We have entered an era of renewed interest in possible cofactors or predisposing traits for alcoholic cardiomyopathy. In this context, it is appropriate to consider further the arsenic and cobalt beer drinker episodes and thiamine (cocarboxylase) deficiency—or beri-beri heart disease.

## Arsenic-Beer Drinkers' Disease

In 1900 an epidemic (>6000 cases with 70+ deaths) in and near Manchester, England, proved to be due to arsenic-contaminated beer. The illness was characterized by skin, neurological, and gastrointestinal signs and symptoms, as well as prominent cardiovascular manifestations, especially heart failure. Included in a superb clinical description [14] were the following: (a) "cases were associated with so much heart failure and so little pigmentation that they were diagnosed as beri-beri...;" (b) "so great has been the cardiac muscle failure that...the principal cause of death has been cardiac failure...;" and (c) "at postmortem examinations the only prominent signs were the interstitial nephritis and the dilated flabby heart..."

Over the next few years there were lively entries in *The Lancet* that alluded to a possible earlier French outbreak due to wine contaminated by chemicals used to treat cane sugar. It was estimated that the affected beer had 2-4 parts per million of arsenic, an amount not, in itself, likely to cause serious toxicity. Gowers [15] mentioned that he prescribed 10 times the amount of arsenic involved for epilepsy over long periods of time with no toxicity; thus "the amount of arsenic...was not sufficient to explain the poisoning." Some persons seemed to have a "peculiar idiosyncrasy," in that "many persons became ill who drank less beer than others not affected." A report by an appointed committee [16] suggested that "alcohol predisposed people to arsenic poisoning." As best one can determine, no one suggested the converse.

## Cobalt-Beer Drinkers' Disease

Sometimes, history repeats itself. Recognized sixty-five years after the arsenic-beer episode, this condition was similar in some respects. In the mid-1960s reports appeared of epidemics of heart failure among beer drinkers in Omaha and Minneapolis in the United States , Quebec in Canada, and Leuven, Belgium. The condition developed fairly abruptly in chronic heavy beer drinkers. The North American patients suffered a high mortality rate, but those who recovered did well despite return, by many, to previous beer habits. The Belgian cases were less acute in onset, longer in duration, and had a lower mortality.

The explanation proved to be the addition of small amounts of cobalt chloride by certain breweries to improve the foaming qualities of beer. Widespread use of detergents (new at that time) in taverns had a depressant effect upon foaming. This etiology was tracked down largely by Quebec investigators [17], and the condition became justly known as Quebec beer-drinkers cardiomyopathy. The largest Quebec brewery had added cobalt to all beer, not only draft beer. Removal of the cobalt additive ended the epidemic in all locations.

In Belgium, where the cobalt concentrations were less and the cardiac manifestations less severe, there were more of the usual findings of chronic cobalt use, such as polycythemia and goiter. However, even in Quebec, where cobalt doses were greatest, 12 liters of contaminated beer provided only about 8 mg of cobalt, less than 20% of the dose sometimes used as a hematinic. The hematinic use had not been implicated as a cause of heart disease, whereas the first cases of this dramatic heart condition occurred 4-8 weeks after cobalt was added to beer,

Thus it was established that both cobalt and substantial amounts of alcohol seemed needed to produce this condition. Most exposed persons did not develop the condition. Despite much speculation, biochemical mechanisms were not established. One observer [18] summed up the arsenic and cobalt episodes thus: "This is the second known metal induced cardiotoxic syndrome produced by contaminated beer."

The arsenic and cobalt episodes raise, by analogy, consideration of other cofactors in alcoholic cardiomyopathy; possibilities include cardiotropic viruses, drugs, selenium, copper, and iron. Deficiencies (zinc, magnesium, protein, and vitamins) have also been suggested as cofactors, but deficiency of thiamine is probably the only one with solid proof of cardiac malfunction.

## Cardiovascular Beriberi

Aalsmeer and Wenckebach's classical description [11] defined, in Javanese polished-rice eaters, high-output heart failure resulting from decreased peripheral vascular resistance. Thus, many assumed that heart failure among Western heavy alcohol drinkers was due to associated nutritional deficiency states. A few heart failure cases in North American and European alcoholics suited this hypothesis. Most did not, however, as they had low output heart failure, were well-nourished, and responded poorly to thiamine. Chronicity of the condition, with ultimate irreversibility was used by some to explain the situation. Blacket and Palmer [19] stated the following view: "It (beri-beri) responds completely to thiamine, but merges imperceptibly into another disease, called alcoholic cardiomyopathy, which doesn't respond to thiamine." It is now established that, in beriberi, there is generalized peripheral arteriolar dilatation creating, effectively, a large arteriovenous shunt and high resting cardiac output. A few cases of complete recovery with thiamine within 1-2 weeks have been documented.

Thus, many cases earlier called "cardiovascular beriberi" would now be called "alcoholic heart disease." Does chronic thiamine deficiency play a role in some cases of alcoholic cardiomyopathy? Currently unpopular, this hypothesis has not been proved or disproved.

**Hypertension**

Lian [20] reported a threshold relationship between heavy drinking and hypertension (HTN) in WWI middle-aged French servicemen. Unless Dr. Lian's French soldiers exaggerated, they were prodigious drinkers, as the HTN threshold appeared at $\geq 2$ liters/wine per day. There was an almost 60-year lapse before further attention was paid to this subject. Starting in the mid-1970s, dozens of cross-sectional and prospective epidemiologic studies have solidly established an empiric alcohol-HTN link [21-22]. These studies involve both sexes and various ages and include North American, European, Australian, and Japanese populations, with an apparent threshold amount of drinking associated with higher blood pressure at approximately 3 drinks/day. Most studies show no increased HTN with lighter drinking; several show an unexplained J-shaped curve in women with lowest pressures in lighter drinkers. There seems to be independence from adiposity, salt intake, education, smoking, beverage type (wine, liquor, or beer), and several other potential confounders.

Clinical experiments of the alcohol/HTN relationship first showed [23] in hospitalized hypertensive men that 3-4 days of drinking 4 pints of beer raised blood pressure and that 3-4 days of abstinence resulted in lower pressures, with pressure changes occurring in several days to a week. Neither these nor later experiments confirmed an increased pressure related to acute alcohol withdrawal. Similar results were later seen in ambulatory normotensives and hypertensives [21]. Other interventional studies have shown that heavier alcohol intake interferes with drug treatment of HTN and that moderation or avoidance of alcohol improves the effectiveness of other nonpharmacologic interventions such as weight reduction, exercise, or sodium restriction [21]. Even in the absence of an established mechanism, the intervention studies strongly support a causal hypothesis. It now seems probable that alcohol restriction might play a major role in HTN management and prevention.

## Arrhythmias

The concept of the "holiday heart phenomenon" was based on the observation [24], that supraventricular arrhythmias in alcoholics without overt cardiomyopathy were most likely to occur on Mondays or between Christmas and New Year's Day. An association of heavier alcohol consumption with atrial arrhythmias had been suspected for decades, perhaps occurring especially after a large meal accompanied with much alcohol. Some have suggested that atrial flutter was especially likely to be so associated, but various atrial arrhythmias have been reported to be associated with spree drinking. Atrial fibrillation is the commonest manifestation. With or without specific treatment, the problem typically resolves with abstinence. A Kaiser Permanente study [25] compared atrial arrhythmias in 1,322 persons reporting 6+ drinks per day to arrhythmias in 2,644 light drinkers. There was, at least, a doubled relative risk in the heavier drinkers for atrial fibrillation, atrial flutter, supraventricular tachycardia, and atrial premature complexes.

## Stroke

Imprecise diagnosis of stroke type prior to modern imaging techniques plagued earlier studies of relationships of alcohol drinking to stroke. All studies of alcohol and stroke, old and new, are greatly complicated by the complex and disparate relationships of both stroke and alcohol to other cardiovascular conditions. Furthermore, some studies examined only drinking sprees; some others did not differentiate between hemorrhagic and ischemic strokes. Several reports suggested that alcohol use, especially heavier drinking, was associated with higher risk of stroke [26].

There is some consensus that heavier drinkers are at higher risk of hemorrhagic stroke. Several recent studies suggest that regular lighter drinkers may also be at higher risk of hemorrhagic stroke types, but at lower risk of several types of ischemic stroke [26].

At this time there is no consensus about the relations of alcohol drinking to the various types of cerebrovascular disease and agreement only that more study of this important subject is needed.

## Coronary Heart Disease

"Wine and spirituous liquors...afford considerable relief'
William Heberden, 1786

After this classic description of angina pectoris [27], it was widely presumed that alcohol is a coronary vasodilator [28-29]. However, data from exercise ECG tests [30-31] suggest that alcohol does not improve myocardial oxygen deficiency and that symptomatic benefit is purely subjective and likely to be dangerously misleading in patients with angina. There are very inadequate data suggesting any major immediate effect of alcohol upon coronary blood flow [32-33]. In the first half of the 1900s there were reports of an apparent inverse relationship between alcohol consumption and atherosclerotic disease, including CHD [34-37]. One explanation put forward was that premature deaths in heavier drinkers precluded development of CHD [38-39]. Since 1974 a number of population and case-control studies have solidly established an inverse relationship between alcohol drinking and either fatal or nonfatal CHD. Data that support the existence of plausible protective mechanisms against CHD by alcohol have also appeared [32-33]. Thus, it now seems likely that alcohol drinking protects against CHD.

In 1819 Dr. Samuel Black, an Irish physician with a great interest in angina pectoris and of considerable perception with respect to epidemiologic aspects, wrote what is probably the first commentary pertinent to the "French Paradox." He noted much angina in Ireland, but lack of discussion of the condition by French physicians, whom he greatly respected. His interpretation of the disparity in CHD between Ireland and France was noteworthy [40]. He attributed the low angina prevalence in France to "the French habits and modes of living, coinciding with the benignity of their climate and the peculiar character of their moral affections." It was to be 160 years before data were presented from the first international comparison study to suggest less CHD in wine drinking countries than in beer or liquor drinking countries [41]. There are now several confirmatory international comparison studies as well as reports of nonalcohol antioxidant phenolic compounds or antithrombotic substances in wine, especially red wine [32-33]. However, prospective population studies show no consensus about the wine/liquor/beer issue [42-43]. This question remains unresolved at this time.

## The J-Shaped Alcohol-Mortality Curve

One report of the J-curve (lighter drinkers at lowest risk, heavier drinkers at highest risk) alcohol-mortality phenomenon preceded other population study reports by half a century. A Baltimore investigator [44] described this relationship in a study of 5,248 tuberculosis patients and controls. "Heavy/steady" drinkers had the highest mortality; "abstainers" were next; and "moderate" drinkers had the lowest mortality. In the absence of an explanation, and in U.S. Prohibition days, his interpretation was predictably cautious. He concluded that moderate drinking was "not harmful." Perhaps his major contribution was to realize the fallacy in comparing all drinkers to abstainers, which masks the J-curve. He said, "one cannot judge the role of diet by starvation or excess."

## The "Sensible Drinking Limit"

Attempts to define a safe limit are not a new phenomenon, since the medical risks of heavier drinking and the relative safety of lighter drinking have long been evident. Probably the most famous such limit has been known for more than 100 years as "Anstie's Rule" [45]. This suggested an upper limit of approximately three standard drinks daily. Although this limit was intended to apply primarily to mature men, Sir Anstie was a distinguished neurologist and public health activist who emphasized individual variability in the ability to handle alcohol. Considerations of individual risks and benefits should be a major focus of any discussion [45] and becomes the primary consideration when a health practitioner advises his or her client. Several contemporary data-based definitions are similar to Sir Anstie's common- sense-based concept.

## References

1.  Klatsky AL. Cardiovascular effects of alcohol. Scientific American Sci and Med 1995;2: 28-37.
2.  Friedreich N. Handbuch der speziellen Pathologic und Therapie. 5th Sect. Krankheiten des Herzens. Erlangen: Ferdinand Enke, 1861.
3.  Walsche WH. Diseases of the heart and great vessels. 4th ed. London: Smith, Elder, 1873
4.  Strumpel A. A textbook of medicine. New York: Appleton, 1890:294.
5.  Steell G. Heart failure as a result of chronic alcoholism. Med Chron (Manchester) 1893; 18:1-22.
6.  Osler W. The principles and practice of medicine. 3rd ed. New York: Appleton, 1899.
7.  Bollinger O. Ueber die Haussigkeit und Ursachen der idiopathischen Herzhypertrophie in München. Disch Med Wochenschr (Stuttgart) 1884;10:180.
8.  Steell G. Textbook on diseases of the heart. Philadelphia: Blakiston, 1902:79.
9.  MacKenzie J. The study of the pulse. Edinburgh: Y.J. Pentland, 1906:237.
10. Vaquez H. Maladies du coeur, Bailliere et Fils, Paris, 1921.
11. Aalsmeer WC, Wenckebach KF. Herz und Kreislauf bei der Beri-Beri Krankheit. Arch Int Med (Vienna) 1929;16:193-272.
12. Keefer CS. The beri-beri heart. Arch Intern Med 1930;45:1-22.
13. Urbano-Marquez A, Estrich R, Navarro-Lopez F, Grau JM, Mont L, Rubin E. The effects of alcoholism on skeletal and cardiac muscle. N Engl J Med 1989;320:409-15.
14. Reynolds ES. An account of the epidemic outbreak of arsenical poisoning occurring in beer drinkers in the north of England and the Midland Counties in 1900. Lancet 1901;I: 166-70.
15. Gowers WR. In: Royal Medical and Chirugical Society. Epidemic of arsenical poisoning in beer-drinkers in the north of England during the year 1900. Lancet 1901;I:98-100.
16. Royal Commission Appointed to Inquire into Arsenical Poisoning from the Consumption of Beer and other Articles of Food or Drink. Final report. Part I. London: Wyman and Sons, 1903.
17. Morin Y, Daniel P. Quebec beer-drinkers' cardiomyopathy: Etiologic considerations. Can Med Assoc J 1967;97:926-28.
18. Alexander CS. Cobalt and the heart. Ann Intern Med 1969;70:411-13.
19. Blacket RB, Palmer AJ. Haemodynamic studies in high output beri-beri. Br Heart J 1960; 22:483-501.
20. Lian C. L'alcoholisme cause d'hypertension arterielle. Bull Acad Med (Paris) 1915:74:525-28.
21. Beilin LJ, Puddey IB. Alcohol and hypertension. Clin Exp Hypertens Theory Pract 1992; A14(1,2):119-38.
22. Klatsky AL. Blood pressure and alcohol intake. In: Laragh JH, Brenner BM., editors. Hypertension: Pathophysiology, diagnosis, and management. 2nd ed. New York: Raven

Press, Ltd., 1995:2649-67.

23.    Potter JF, Beevers DG. Pressor effect of alcohol in hypertension. Lancet 1984;1:119-22.
24.    Ettinger PO, Wu CF, De La Cruz C, Weisse AB, Ahmed SS, Regan TJ. Arrhythmias and the "holiday heart": Alcohol-associated cardiac rhythm disorders. Am Heart J 1978;95: 555-62.
25.    Cohen EJ, Klatsky AL, Armstrong MA. Alcohol use and supraventricular arrhythmia. Am J Cardiol 1988;62:971-73.
26.    Van Gign J, Stampfer MJ, Wolfe C, Algra A. The association between alcohol consumption and stroke. In: Health issues related to alcohol consumption. Verschuren PM, editor. Washington DC, ILSI Press:1993: 43-80.
27.    Heberden W. Some account of a disorder of the breast. Med Trans R Coll Physicians (London) 1786;2:59-67.
28.    White PD. Heart disease. New York: Macmillan, 1931: 436.
29.    Levine SA. In: Clinical heart disease. 4th ed. Philadelphia: Saunders, 1951: 98.
30.    Russek, HI, Naegele, CF, Regan, FD. Alcohol in the treatment of angina pectoris J Am Med Assoc 1950;143:355-57.
31.    Orlando J, Aronow, WS, Cassidy J, Prakash, R. Effect of ethanol on angina pectoris. Ann Intern Med 1976;84:652-55.
32.    Renaud S, Criqui MH, Farchi G, Veenstra J. Alcohol drinking and coronary heart disease. In: Health issues related to alcohol consumption. Verschuren PM, editor. Washington DC, ILSI Press 1993:81-124.
33.    Klatsky AL. Epidemiology of coronary heart disease--Influence of alcohol. Alcohol Clin Exp Res 1994;18:88-96.
34.    Cabot RC. The relation of alcohol to arteriosclerosis. J Am Med Assoc 1904;43:774-75.
35.    Hultgen JF. Alcohol and nephritis: Clinical study of 460 cases of chronic alcoholism. J Am Med Assoc 1910;55:279-81.
36.    Leary T. Therapeutic value of alcohol, with special consideration of relations of alcohol to cholesterol, and thus to diabetes, to arteriosclerosis, and to gallstones. N Engl J Med 1931;205:231-42.
37.    Wilens SL. The relationship of chronic alcoholism to atherosclerosis. J Am Med Assoc 1947;135:1136-39.
38.    Ruebner BH, Miyai K, Abbey H. The low incidence of myocardial infarction in hepatic cirrhosis - a statistical artefact? Lancet 1961;ii:1435-36.
39.    Parrish HM, Eberly AL, Jr. Negative association of coronary atherosclerosis with liver cirrhosis and chronic alcoholism - a statistical fallacy. J Indiana State Med Assoc 1961;54: 341-47.
40.    Black S. Clinical and pathological reports. Newry: Alex Wilkinson, 1819:1-47.
41.    St. Leger AS, Cochrane AL, Moore F. Factors associated with cardiac mortality in developed countries with particular reference to the consumption of wine. Lancet 1979;1: 1017-20.
42.    Rimm E, Klatsky AL, Grobbee D, Stampfer MJ. Review of moderate alcohol consumption and reduced risk of coronary heart disease: Is the effect due to beer, wine, or spirits? BMJ 1996;312:731-36.
43.    Klatsky AL, Armstrong, MA, Friedman GD. Red wine, white wine, liquor, beer, and risk for coronary artery disease hospitalization. Am J Cardiol 1997;80:416-20.
44.    Pearl R. Alcohol and longevity. New York: Knopf, 1926.

45.    Anstie FE. On the uses of wines in health and disease. New York: JS Redfield, 1870:11-13.

# EFFECTS OF ALCOHOL ON LIPIDS AND LIPOPROTEIN METABOLISM

Jean-Charles Fruchart, François Cambien, and Patrick Duriez

## Introduction

The health effects of alcohol consumption remain complex for several reasons: the risks and benefits accrue over many years; assessment of drinking is generally based on self-report; drinking habits change over time; and studies which estimate average daily drinking disregard how or when the beverage was consumed. In addition, alcohol consumption is associated with lifestyle factors which may confound relationship with disease. Research into the effect of alcohol on cardiovascular disease has indicated protective effects from moderate consumption (1-2 drinks a day) [1]. Recent studies reinforce the consistent finding of a J-shaped inverse association between alcohol and cardiovascular disease morbidity and mortality, primarily as a result of the association between alcohol and coronary heart disease [2]. Analyses of potential mediators of effects of alcohol on cardiovascular disease show that it increases high density lipoprotein (HDL)-cholesterol levels and favorably influences thrombotic factors, especially fibrinogen, and also fibrinolytic factors. Some evidence also suggests moderate alcohol consumption may reduce insulin resistance [3]. However, studies also show an adverse effect of alcohol, particularly at higher doses, on blood pressure (leading to hypertension) and directly on the myocardium (leading to arrhythmias and myocardiopathy). In central and eastern Europe and the former Soviet Union, a growing body of epidemiological research indicates a positive rather than negative association between alcohol consumption and cardiovascular deaths, especially sudden cardiac deaths [4]. Furthermore, epidemiological evidence indicate that recent heavy alcohol consumption increases the risk for all major types of stroke [5].

Alcoholic fatty liver and hyperlipemia result from the interaction of ethanol and its oxidation products with hepatic lipid metabolism. An early target of ethanol toxicity is mitochondrial fatty acid oxidation. Acetaldehyde and reactive oxygen species have been incriminated in the pathogenesis of the mitochondrial injury. Microsomal changes offset deleterious accumulation of fatty acids, leading to enhanced formation of triacyglycerols, which are partly secreted into the plasma and partly accumulate in the liver. Alcoholic hyperlipemia results primarily from increased hepatic secretion of very low density lipoprotein (VLDL) and secondarily from impairment in the removal of triacylglycerol-rich

11

R. Paoletti et al. (eds.), Moderate Alcohol Consumption and Cardiovascular Disease, 11–22.

lipoproteins from the plasma. Hyperlipemia tends to disappear because of enhanced lipolytic activity and aggravation of the liver injury [6]. With moderate alcohol consumption, the increase in HDL becomes the predominant feature. Its mechanism is multifactorial (increased hepatic secretion and increased extrahepatic formation as well as decreased removal) and explains part of the enhanced cholesterol transport from tissues to bile. Since the initial observation by Miller and Miller [7], many epidemiological studies have demonstrated the inverse correlation between the concentration of HDL-cholesterol and the risk of myocardial infarction. Therefore, increase in HDL-cholesterol plasma levels with moderate alcohol consumption might contribute to, but not fully account for, the effects on atherosclerosis and/or coronary heart disease attributed to moderate drinking. The paper will focus on the effects of alcohol on HDL and apolipoprotein A-I- and A-II-containing lipoprotein particles.

## HDL Metabolism in Plasma

HDL is the most malleable of lipoprotein species since all of its components undergo rapid interparticle exchange. It is composed of a number of subspecies (pre-beta HDL, $HDL_2$, and $HDL_3$) whose interconversions are governed by the exchange and lipolysis mechanisms as well as by the action of the enzyme lecithin:cholesterol acyl transferase (LCAT). The role of HDL is believed to be that of a cellular cholesterol acceptor which removes excess sterol from cell surfaces and traps it in the form of cholesteryl ester in the lipoprotein transport system. A gradient of reverse cholesterol transport is maintained, either by the liver taking up cholesteryl-ester-laden HDL or by transfer via cholesteryl-ester transfer protein (CETP) of HDL cholesteryl ester to apolipoprotein B-containing particles, which are themselves subject to rapid uptake by the liver.

Mature HDL in plasma exists in two major density classes, $HDL_2$ and $HDL_3$, which can be subdivided further on the basis of apo A composition. Twenty years ago [8], immunological methods revealed that HDL are a heterogeneous mixture of particles comprising two major classes of apo A-I containing particles: LpA-I:A-II, particles containing both apo A-I and apo A-II and LpA-I, particles containing apo A-I but not apo A-II.

## Physiological Roles of LpA-I and LpA-I:A-II

LpA-I and LpA-I:A-II differ in their physiological roles, particularly in their capacity in inducing cellular cholesterol efflux and in removing excess cholesterol from cell surfaces. Long-term exposure of cholesterol-preloaded adipose cells (Ob17) to LpA-I particles promoted cholesterol efflux. Such efflux was not observed in the presence of LpA-I:A-II [9]. Huang et al. [10] confirm that LpA-I was more effective than LpA-I:A-II in both uptake and esterification of fibroblast-derived cholesterol. Nevertheless, different studies reported that both LpA-I and LpA-I:A-II demonstrate equal ability to promote efflux of cholesterol from several types of cells, such as fibroblasts, smooth muscle cells, and

Fu5AH [11,12]. Evidence has emerged that the metabolism of LpA-I and LpA-I:A-II particles occurs by distinct pathways [13,14,15]. Rader et al. [14] have shown that apo A-I on LpA-I is catabolized faster than apo A-I on Lp A-I:A-II. Triglyceride, LpA-I, and LpA-I:A-II concentrations correlated with HDL-cholesterol in normolipidemic men, but there was no correlation between apo A-I-containing particles and plasma triglyceride level [16].

## Clinical Significance of LpA-I and LpA-I:A-II

The clinical significance of particles differentiated by apolipoprotein content is not entirely clear. LpA-I, but not LpA-I:A-II, was found to be lower in normolipidemic patients with angiographically documented coronary heart disease, compared to asymptomatic subjects and a group of patients with angiographically normal coronary arteries [17]. However, in a study which found triglyceride levels to be higher in the patients than in the controls, both LpA-I and LpA-I:A-II were reduced to a similar degree in patients with coronary heart disease [18]. O'Brien et al. [19] also reported that LpA-I and LpA-I:A-II were similarly reduced in subjects with coronary disease.

The android pattern of body fat distribution has been shown to increase the risk of metabolic and coronary heart disease. In obese normolipidaemic, nondiabetic, nonsmoker subjects over 18 years old body mass index (BMI) was not correlated with protective lipid parameters but only with triglycerides while waist-hip ratio (WHR) was inversely correlated with LpA-I and HDL-cholesterol. After adjustment, LpA-I was lower in men and in upper body obese women and was a better indicator of body fat distribution than HDL-cholesterol or apo A-I [20].

The high incidence and prevalence of coronary heart disease in diabetes mellitus is clearly established. Brites et al. [21] showed that HDL-cholesterol and apo A-I were significantly decreased in type 2 diabetic patients due to a selective reduction in LpA-I subfraction.

## The Role of LpA-I and LpA-I: A-II in Atherosclerosis Development in Transgenic Animal Models

Transgenic animal models (mice [22,23,24] and rabbits [25]) clearly demonstrate that overexpression of human apo A-I leading to a high concentration of HDL particles containing mainly apo A-I rich HDL (LpA-I) inhibits atherosclerosis development when the plasma is rich in apo B-containing particles. On the other hand, the role of apo A-II is not clearly demonstrated. Some studies [24] have suggested that the transgenesis of apo A-II increases atherogenesis and that apo A-II rich HDL are atherogenic while apo A-I/apo A-II HDL (LpA-I:A-II) are poorly antiatherogenic in comparison with apo A-I rich HDL (LpA-I). These animal models suggest that lipoprotein particle mimicking what is called LpA-I in human clinical studies are highly antiatherogenic while the role of LpA-I:A-II is not clearly demonstrated and depend on other metabolic factors.

## Effect of Alcohol Consumption on HDL-, HDL$_2$-, HDL$_3$-Cholesterol Plasma Levels

Moderate, heavy, and addictive alcohol consumption differently alter lipoprotein plasma levels. Seppa et al. [26] studied serum lipid values in 380 men, including controls (teetotalers and moderate drinkers), heavy drinkers, and alcoholics. Total cholesterol was higher in heavy drinkers (244 mg/dL) than in controls (232 mg/dL) while it was lower in alcoholics (210 mg/dL); on the other hand HDL-cholesterol was higher in alcoholics (64 mg/dL) and in heavy drinkers (48 mg/dL) than in controls (44 mg/dL). Accordingly, there was a highly significant difference in the HDL-cholesterol/total cholesterol ratio between alcoholics and controls (0.32 versus 0.19, respectively) but there was no significant difference in this ratio between controls and heavy drinkers or between teetotalers and moderate drinkers. Therefore, moderate alcohol intake apparently does not change HDL-cholesterol/total cholesterol ratio. This data suggests that if moderate drinking is protective against coronary heart disease, the mechanism is independent of the ratio "antiatherogenic-cholesterol"/total cholesterol.

Sillanaukee et al. [27] studied the relationship of alcohol consumption to changes in HDL-subfractions. Serum total HDL-cholesterol and its HDL$_2$ and HDL$_3$ subfractions were blindly compared between consecutive middle-aged men (teetotallers, moderate drinkers, heavy drinkers) participating in a voluntary health screaning and in male alcoholics. Alcohol consumption correlated significantly with total-cholesterol, HDL$_2$, and HDL$_3$ when all subjects were included but the correlation disappeared when alcoholics were excluded. In comparison with teetotallers, alcoholics had significantly higher total HDL-cholesterol, HDL$_2$, and HDL$_3$ values. Moderate or heavy intake of alcohol had no effect on HDL$_2$ but increased the HDL$_3$ fraction. This data suggests that if moderate alcohol consumption is mediated by HDL, it may not be accounted for by changes in the HDL$_2$ fraction. The observed increases in the concentration of the HDL$_3$ fraction, however, suggest that this subfraction may not be inert with respect to coronary disease and could have a role in the protective effect.

## Effects of Alcohol Withdrawal on HDL-, HDL$_2$, HDL$_3$ Cholesterol Plasma Levels

Alcohol withdrawal induced a significant decrease in HDL-cholesterol and apo A-I in chronic alcoholic subjects [28]. HDL-cholesterol and apo A-I showed a biphasic variation with significant postwithdrawal changes which became less pronounced after 6 months of abstinence. A 38% decrease in mean total HDL-cholesterol levels was noted by Lamisse et al. [29] after withdrawal therapy in alcoholic men, and this was due mainly to a drop in HDL$_3$-cholesterol concentrations (-43%), although the decrease in HDL$_2$-cholesterol concentrations was also significant (-21%) but less marked. These results were not dependent on quantities of alcohol ingested before therapy and on duration of hospitalization, while the magnitude of the apo A-I decrease after alcohol withdrawal was positively related to the duration of hospitalization.

## Effects of Alcohol Consumption on LpA-I and LpA-I:A-II Plasma Levels

In 1990 we investigated the relationships between LpA-I and LpA-I:A-II concentrations and alcohol consumption in 344 men and found that LpA-I-A-II increased and LpA-I levels decreased with an increasing alcohol intake [30].

Nevertheless, recent data showed that alcohol consumption induces significant increases in both LpA-I and LpA-I:A-II plasma levels:

- 615 control subjects of the ECTIM Study [31] were distribute in five groups of alcohol consumption: nondrinkers; 0 < or < 15 g/day, 15 < or 36 g/day, 36 < or < 66 g/day and > 66 g/day. After adjustment for age, BMI, cigarette consumption, and country (France and Northern Ireland), alcohol consumption was associated with an increase in HDL-cholesterol (47 mg/dL [nondrinkers] versus 59 mg/dL [> 66 g/day]), apolipoprotein A-I (137 mg/dL [nondrinkers] versus 160 mg/dL [> 66 g/day]); apolipoprotein A-II (32 mg/dL [nondrinkers] versus 41 mg/dl [> 66 g/day]), LpA-I (46 mg/dL [nondrinkers] versus 50 mg/dL [> 66 g/day]), LpA-I:A-II (75 mg/dL [nondrinkers] versus 91 mg/dL [> 66 g/day]).

- Branchi et al. [32] have shown that both LpA-I and LpA-I:A-II were significantly higher in men drinking more than 30 g a day of alcohol than in nondrinkers (LpA-I: difference between means 6.5 mg/dL; LpA-I:A-II: difference between means 11.5 mg/dL). The association of alcohol consumption with LpA-I and LpA-I:A-II levels was independent from age, BMI, physical activity, serum triglycerides, and diet composition.

- Lecomte et al. [33] also reported that alcohol consumption increases both types of apolipoprotein A-I particles. In 132 healthy subjects, including 55 low drinkers (< 20 g/day), 36 moderate drinkers (20-50 g/day), and 41 heavy drinkers (> 50 g/day), and in 97 hospitalized alcoholic patients (> 100 g/day) without severe liver disease, before and after 21 days of withdrawal treatment. Serum concentrations of apo A-I, LpA-I, and LpA-I:A-II increased significantly with alcohol intake (low drinkers versus alcoholics: apo A-I: 145 mg/dL versus 178 mg/dL; LpA-I: 45 mg/dL versus 56 mg/dL; LpA-I:A-II: 99 mg/dL versus 122 mg/dL, respectively). After withdrawal, the concentrations of serum apo A-I, LpA-I and LpA-I:A-II decreased significantly, reaching values comparable with those in low drinkers. In multiple regression analysis, alcohol consumption remained positively correlated to apo A-I and LpA-I:A-II concentrations. Although the increase of antiatherogenic apolipoproteins and lipoproteins (and the decrease of those known to be atherogenic) were generally marked in alcoholics, alcohol-related modifications of these markers were very limited in these French healthy men. Authors concluded that moderate alcohol consumption (20-50 g/day) is unlikely to protect against ischemic heart disease through an effect on the proteins measured in this study.

- Valimaki et al. [34] studied the effects of alcohol consumption and alcohol withdrawal on apo A-I containing particles in alcoholic women. On admission the apo A-II concentration was increased by 48% and it was normalized during abstention. Among apo A-I containing lipoproteins the most prominent change occurred in LpA-I:A-II, which fell by 32 % during 1 week of alcohol withdrawal. In contrast to alcoholic men, there was no significant elevation of $HDL_3$ cholesterol and apo A-I.

- Recently, we have investigated the relationship between apolipoprotein A-I containing lipoprotein fractions and environmental factors in the Prospective Epidemiological Study of Myocardial Infarction (PRIME study) [35]. Between 1991 and 1993, 10,596 subjects (50-59 year-old males, free of diabetes mellitus, of cardiovascular disease, of hypertriglyceridemia or taking antihypertensive or hypolipemic drugs) were recruited. The analysis included 2,059 subjects in Toulouse (France); 2,076 in Strasbourg (France); 1,963 in Lille (France); and 2,259 in Belfast (Northern Ireland). Moderate alcohol consumption (10 g/day) increased apo A-I, LpA-I, and LpA-I:A-II by 1.39, 0.21, and 1.21 mg/dL, respectively. This effect remained virtually unchanged by simultaneous adjustment for BMI, WHR, cigarette smoking, physical activity, and triglycerides. Moreover, the effect of alcohol on apo A-I and LpA-I:A-II remained significantly positive, if attenuated after adjustment for HDL cholesterol. Conversely, the relationship between LpA-I and alcohol consumption disappeared after adjustment for HDL cholesterol.

## Mechanisms of the Positive Relationship Between Alcohol Intake and Plasma Concentrations of HDL-Cholesterol, LpA-I, and LpA-I:A-II

### APO A-I AND APO A-II METABOLISM

We have measured [36] apo A-I and apo A-II in HDL after endogenous labelling using amino acid labelled with stable isotope in normolipidemic healthy volunteers at the end of two consecutive 4-week period, one without alcohol and the other with an intake of 50 g/day of alcohol (red wine). Cholesterol, triglycerides did not vary significantly during the two periods, whereas HDL cholesterol increased from 43.8 to 50 mg/dL. Apo A-I and apo A-II increased significantly (20% and 60%, respectively) after the diet was supplemented with alcohol. LpA-I:A-II increased from 73.8 to 101.6 mg/dL (+32%), whereas alcohol had no effect on the concentration of LpA-I. The alcohol treatment did not significantly alter the metabolism of apo A-I. Conversely, the fractional catabolic rate of apo A-II decreased significantly by 21% with alcohol, whereas the production rate of apo A-II tended to increase by 18%. Therefore, the decrease in the fractional catabolic rate of apo A-II could lead to an accumulation of apo A-II containing lipoproteins in plasma and account for the dramatic increase in LpA-I:A-II observed in the plasma of subjects consuming alcohol.

## CHOLESTERYL-ESTER METABOLISM

Triglyceride from chylomicrons and VLDL is transferred into HDL via cholesteryl-ester transfer protein (CETP). The triglyceride-enriched $HDL_2$ so formed are then hydrolyzed by hepatic lipase (HL) to form $HDL_3$. $HDL_3$ is postulated to be converted back into $HDL_2$ by the acquisition of phospholipids and free cholesterol shed from lipolyzed VLDL and chylomicrons, and the subsequent action of lecithin-cholesterol acyl transferase (LCAT). The validity of the exchange/lipolysis cycle in controlling HDL *in vivo* is demonstrated by examining the characteristics of HDL in a number of human deficiency states. In abetalipoproteinemia, where there are no triglyceride-rich lipoproteins to act as donors, HDL exists mainly as cholesteryl ester-rich $HDL_2$. Similarly, subjects with inherited CETP deficiency have high levels of cholesteryl-rich $HDL_2$. Lack of HL leads to a condition in which $HDL_2$ is the major, if not only, HDL species. These natural experiments are now supplemented by seminal studies in transgenic animals, in which it has been shown that possession of the human apo A-I, C-III, and CETP genes is sufficient to cause expression of a high plasma triglyceride/low-HDL phenotype in mice [37]. A number of genetic studies have shown that polymorphisms at the CETP [38,39] and HL loci [40] can markedly influence HDL cholesterol levels.

A polymorphism of CETP gene (CETP/TaqIB) with two alleles B1 (60%) and B2 (40%) has been investigated in relation to lipid variables and the risk of myocardial infarction in a large case control study (ECTIM) of men aged 25-64 [41]. No association was observed between the polymorphism and LDL or VLDL related to lipid variables. Conversely, B2 carriers had reduced levels of plasma CETP and increased levels of HDL-cholesterol. The effects of the polymorphism on plasma CETP and HDL-cholesterol were independent, suggesting the presence of at least two functional variants linked to B2. A search for these variants on the coding sequence of the CETP gene failed to identify them. The effect of B2 on plasma HDL-cholesterol was absent in subjects drinking < 25 g/day of alcohol but increased commensurably, with higher values of alcohol consumption. A similar interaction was not observed for plasma CETP. The odds-ratio for myocardial infarction of B2 homozygotes decreased from 1.0 in nondrinkers to 0.34 in those drinking 75 g/day or more.

The effect of the CETP 1405V polymorphism on plasma lipids was investigated in healthy Icelandic men and women [42]. The V allele frequency was 0.31 in this population. Men (but not in women) who were homozygous for the V405 allele had 9% higher apo A-I and 14% higher HDL-cholesterol levels than those homozygous for the common I405 allele. Analysis of interaction between the environmental, life-style factors, and genotype in men for the traits of HDL-cholesterol and apo A-I showed statistically significant interaction of the genotype only with alcohol consumption. The nonsmoking men who reported alcohol consumption and who were homozygous for the CETP V405 allele had 16% higher plasma apo A-I concentration than those who carried the I405 allele, and up to 20% higher apo A-I level than smokers. On the basis of prospective studies carried out on the Icelandic population, nonsmoking, alcohol-consuming men who are homozygous for the V405 allele could have from 32% to 40% lower risk of having a heart attack.

Riemens et al. [43] have shown that plasma LCAT, CETP, and phospholipid-transfer protein (PLTP) activities were not related to alcohol consumption while HDL-cholesterol was higher in alcohol consumer, indicating that the higher HDL-cholesterol associated with moderate alcohol consumption is, therefore, unlikely to be caused by an effect on plasma LCAT, CETP, or PLTP activity levels.

## Type of Alcoholic Beverage and HDL-Cholesterol Levels

Despite a high level of risk factors such as cholesterol, diabetes, hypertension, and a high intake of saturated fat, French males display the lowest mortality rate from ischemic disease and cardiovascular diseases in Western industrialized nations (36% lower than the USA and 39% lower than the UK). The French Paradox has led to speculation that wine is the only protective alcoholic beverage for coronary vascular disease, or at least that it has a stronger effect through the action of multiple antioxidants like polyphenols. Nevertheless, recent analysis of the MONICA study clearly demonstrated that the French Paradox was a mirage according to the following arguments: 1) France is geographically situated between northern Europe (with high cardiovascular risk) and southern Europe (with low cardiovascular risk). MONICA's data shows that the French's southern-northern gradient of cardiovascular risk is perfectly inserted, without disruption, into the southern-northern Europe's gradient of cardiovascular diseases: cardiovascular mortalities in the French's border areas being the same than in the neighboring foreigner border areas (ie, northern France like southern Belgium; eastern France like western Germany; southwestern France like northern Spain). 2) In the past, French doctors underdiagnosed coronary heart disease as the cause of death in the death certificates.

Furthermore, although wine does appear more protective in ecological studies, studies within cohorts show similar effects across alcoholic beverages, suggesting confounding in ecological studies by diet, lifestyle, or other variables [3]. The key component of alcoholic beverages thus appears to be ethanol, consistent with the known potent effects of ethanol on HDL cholesterol and thrombotic factors. Gaziano et al. [44] examined the relation of alcoholic beverage type and risk of myocardial infarction in a case-control study among 340 cases of myocardial infarction and an equal number of matched controls. Beer, wine, and liquor drinkers had at least half of their consumption from one beverage type. Compared with nondrinkers, after adjustment for age and sex, reductions in risk of myocardial infarction were similar for regular drinkers of any type of alcoholic beverage (relative risk: 0.54; beer: 0.55; wine: 0.48; liquor: 0.59). HDL-cholesterol levels were significantly higher in all 4 beverage categories when compared with levels in nondrinkers, and adjustment for HDL-cholesterol substantially attenuated the protective effect in all 4 beverages categories. Relative risks were 0.94 for any beverage, 1.09 for beer, 0.97 for wine, and 0.83 for liquor after further adjustment. These data indicate that regular consumption of small to moderate amounts of alcoholic beverages, regardless of the type, reduces the risk of myocardial infarction, and further suggest that there is benefit, in large part, from increases in HDL levels.

## Conclusion

The association between alcohol intake and atherosclerotic cardiovascular disease in epidemiological studies is consistent and shows some protection from cardiovascular disease at consumption levels of one to two drinks a day, but a sharp increase in cardiovascular disease associated with three or more drinks per day [3]. Analyses of potential mediators of effects of alcohol on cardiovascular diseases shows that the main antiatherogenic effect of alcohol might be related to increases in plasma HDL-cholesterol levels. Physiological, clinical, epidemiological, and experimental studies suggest that LpA-I is slightly more active than LpA-I:A-II in inhibiting atherosclerosis development. Low alcohol consumption induces slight increases in HDL-cholesterol, LpA-I, and LpA-I:A-II while high alcohol consumption dramatically induces increases in these lipoprotein fractions. In the majority of the epidemiological and clinical studies alcohol induced higher increases in LpA-I:A-II than in LpA-I. Therefore, alcohol consumption induces increases in both apolipoprotein A-I particles which have been demonstrated as capable in inhibiting atherosclerosis development. These data suggest that slight increases in LpA-I plasma levels at low alcohol consumption might be very active in inhibiting atherosclerosis development.

## References

1.  Zakhari, S, Gordis E. Moderate drinking and cardiovascular health. Proc Assoc Am Physicians 1999;111:148-58.
2.  Sesso HD, Gaziano JM. Alcohol intake and cardiovascular morbidity and mortality. Curr Opin Nephrol Hypertens 1999;8:353-57.
3.  Criqui MH. Do known cardiovascular risk factors mediate the effect of alcohol on cardiovascular disease? Novartis Found Symp 1998;216:159-67; discussion 167-72,159-67.
4.  McKee M, Britton A. the positive relationship between alcohol and heart disease in eastern Europe: Potential physiological mechanisms. J R Soc Med 1998;91:402-7.
5.  Hillbom M, Juvela S, Karttunen V. Mechanisms of alcohol-related strokes. Novartis Found Symp 1998;216:193-204; discussion 204-7, 193-204.
6.  Baraona E, Lieber CS. Alcohol and lipids. Recent Dev Alcohol 1998;14:97-134.
7.  Miller GJ, Miller NE. Plasma-high-density-lipoprotein concentration and development of ischaemic heart-disease. Lancet 1975;1:16-19.
8.  Alaupovic P. The role of apolipoproteins in lipid transport processes. Ric Clin Lab 1982; 12:3-21.
9.  Barkia A, Puchois P, Ghalim N, et al. Differential role of apolipoprotein AI-containing particles in cholesterol efflux from adipose cells. Atherosclerosis 1991;87:135-46.

10.    Huang Y, von Eckardstein A, Wu S, Assmann G. Cholesterol efflux, cholesterol esterification, and cholesteryl ester transfer by LpA-I and LpA-I/A-II in native plasma. Arterioscler Thromb Vasc Biol 1995;15:1412-18.

11.    Oikawa S, Mendez AJ, Cheung MC, Oram JC, Bierman EL. HDL particles in intracellular cholesterol efflux. Circulation 1991;84(Suppl.II):682.

12.    Johnson WJ, Kilsdonk EP, van Tol A, Phillips MC, Rothblat GH. Cholesterol efflux from cells to immunopurified subfractions of human high density lipoprotein: Lp-AI and Lp-AI/AII. J Lipid Res 1991;32:1993-2000.

13.    Rader DJ, Castro G, Zech LA, Fruchart JC, Brewer HB, Jr. In vivo metabolism of apolipoprotein A-I on high density lipoprotein particles LpA-I and LpA-I,A-II. J Lipid Res 1991;32:1849-59.

14.    Rader DJ, Ikewaki K, Duverger N, et al. Markedly accelerated catabolism of apolipoprotein A-II (apoA-II) and high density lipoproteins containing apoA-II in classic lecithin: cholesterol acyltransferase deficiency and fish-eye disease. J Clin Invest 1994; 93:321-30.

15.    James RW, Pometta D. Postprandial lipemia differentially influences high density lipoprotein subpopulations LpAI and LpAI,AII. J Lipid Res 1994;35:1583-91.

16.    Luc G, Parra HJ, Zylberberg G, Fruchart JC. Plasma concentrations of apolipoprotein A-I containing particles in normolipidaemic young men. Eur J Clin Invest 1991;21:118-22.

17.    Puchois P, Kandoussi A, Fievet P, et al. Apolipoprotein A-I containing lipoproteins in coronary artery disease. Atherosclerosis 1987;68:35-40.

18.    Genest JJ, Jr, Bard JM., Fruchart JC, Ordovas JM, Wilson PF, Schaefer EJ. Plasma apolipoprotein A-I, A-II, B, E and C-III containing particles in men with premature coronary artery disease. Atherosclerosis 1991;90:149-57.

19.    O'Brien T, Nguyen TT, Hallaway BJ, et al. The role of lipoprotein A-I and lipoprotein A-I/A-II in predicting coronary artery disease. Arterioscler Thromb Vasc Biol 1995;15:228-31.

20.    Lecerf JM, Masson A, Fruchart JC, Bard JM. Serum Lp AI lipoprotein particles and other antiatherogenic lipid parameters in normolipidaemic obese subjects. Diabetes Metab 1996;22:331-40.

21.    Brites FD, Cavallero E, de Geitere C, et al. Abnormal capacity to induce cholesterol efflux and a new LpA-I pre-beta particle in type 2 diabetic patients. Clin Chim Acta 1999; 279:1-14.

22.    Rubin EM, Krauss RM, Spangler EA, Verstuyft JG, Clift S. M. Inhibition of early atherogenesis in transgenic mice by human apolipoprotein AI. Nature 1991;19:353, 265-67.

23.    Plump AS, Scott CJ, Breslow JL. Human apolipoprotein A-I gene expression increases high density lipoprotein and suppresses atherosclerosis in the apolipoprotein E-deficient mouse. Proc Natl Acad Sci USA 1994;91:9607-11.

24.    Schultz JR, Verstuyft JG, Gong EL, Nichols AV, Rubin EM. Protein composition determines the anti-atherogenic properties of HDL in transgenic mice. Nature 1993;365: 762-64.

25.    Duverger N, Kruth H, Emmanuel F, et al. Inhibition of atherosclerosis development in cholesterol-fed human apolipoprotein A-I-transgenic rabbits. Circulation 1996;94:713-17.

26.    Seppa K, Sillanaukee P, Pitkajarvi T, Nikkila M, Koivula T. Moderate and heavy alcohol consumption have no favorable effect on lipid values [See Comments]. Arch Intern Med

1992;152:297-300.
27.  Sillanaukee P, Koivula T, Jokela H, Myllyharju H, Seppa K. Relationship of alcohol consumption to changes in HDL-subfractions. Eur J Clin Invest 1993;23:486-91.
28.  Wahl D, Paille F. Insulin sensitivity in alcoholics [Letter; Comment]. J Intern Med 1992; 232:288.
29.  Lamisse F, Schellenberg F, Bouyou E, Delarue J, Benard JY, Couet C. Plasma lipids and alcohol consumption in alcoholic men: Effect of withdrawal. Alcohol 1994;29:25-30.
30.  Puchois P, Ghalim N, Zylberberg G, Fievet P, Demarquilly C, Fruchart JC. Effect of alcohol intake on human apolipoprotein A-I-containing lipoprotein subfractions. Arch Intern Med 1990;150:1638-41.
31.  Marques-Vidal P, Cambou JP, Nicaud V, et al. Cardiovascular risk factors and alcohol consumption in France and northern Ireland. Atherosclerosis 1995;115:225-32.
32.  Branchi A, Rovellini A, Tomella C, et al. Association of alcohol consumption with HDL subpopulations defined by apolipoprotein A-I and apolipoprotein A-II content. Eur J Clin Nutr 1997;51:362-65.
33.  Lecomte E, Herbeth B, Paille F, Steinmetz J, Artur Y, Siest G. Changes in serum apolipoprotein and lipoprotein profile induced by chronic alcohol consumption and withdrawal: determinant effect on heart disease? Clin Chem 1996;42:1666-75.
34.  Valimaki M, Kahri J, Laitinen K, et al. High density lipoprotein subfractions, apolipoprotein A-I containing lipoproteins, lipoprotein (a), and cholesterol ester transfer protein activity in alcoholic women before and after ethanol withdrawal. Eur J Clin Invest 1993;23:406-17.
35.  Luc G, Bard JM, Evans A, et al. The relationship between apolipoprotein AI-containing lipoprotein fractions and environmental factors: The prospective epidemiological study of myocardial infarction (PRIME study). Atherosclerosis 2000; in press.
36.  Gottrand F, Beghin L, Duhal N, et al. Moderate red wine consumption in healthy volunteers reduced plasma clearance of apolipoprotein AII. Eur J Clin Invest 1999;29: 387-94.
37.  Hayek T, Azrolan N, Verdery RB, et al. Hypertriglyceridemia and cholesteryl ester transfer protein interact to dramatically alter high density lipoprotein levels, particle sizes, and metabolism. Studies in transgenic mice. J Clin Invest 1993;92:1143-52.
38.  Kondo I, Berg K, Drayna D, Lawn R. DNA polymorphism at the locus for human cholesteryl ester transfer protein (CETP) is associated with high density lipoprotein cholesterol and apolipoprotein levels. Clin Genet 1989;35:49-56.
39.  Freeman DJ, Caslake MJ, Griffin BA, et al. The effect of smoking on post-heparin lipoprotein and hepatic lipase, cholesteryl ester transfer protein and lecithin:cholesterol acyl transferase activities in human plasma. Eur J Clin Invest 1998;28:584-91.
40.  Cohen JC, Wang Z, Grundy SM, Stoesz MR, Guerra R. Variation at the hepatic lipase and apolipoprotein AI/CIII/AIV loci is a major cause of genetically determined variation in plasma HDL cholesterol levels. J Clin Invest 1994;94:2377-84.
41.  Fumeron F, Betoulle D, Luc G, et al. Alcohol intake modulates the effect of a polymorphism of the cholesteryl ester transfer protein gene on plasma high density lipoprotein and the risk of myocardial infarction. J Clin Invest 1995;96:1664-71.
42.  Gudnason V, Thormar K, Humphries SE. Interaction of the cholesteryl ester transfer protein I405V polymorphism with alcohol consumption in smoking and non-smoking healthy men, and the effect on plasma HDL cholesterol and apoAI concentration. Clin

Genet 1997;51:15-21.
43.     Riemens SC, van Tol A, Hoogenberg K, et al. Higher high density lipoprotein cholesterol
        associated with moderate alcohol consumption is not related to altered plasma
        lecithin:cholesterol acyltransferase and lipid transfer protein activity levels. Clin Chim
        Acta 1997;258:105-15.
44.     Gaziano JM, Hennekens CH, Godfried SL, et al. Type of alcoholic beverage and risk of
        myocardial infarction. Am J Cardiol 1999;83:52-57.

# ALCOHOL CONSUMPTION AND CARDIOVASCULAR DISEASE

Michael H. Criqui

## Introduction

The relation of alcohol consumption to cardiovascular disease (CVD) has received intense scientific scrutiny over the past four decades. Although a prodigious amount of data has been collected, no data on CVD outcomes are available from the gold standard for causal interpretation in medical research, the randomized double-blind clinical trial. It is unlikely such a definitive trial will be conducted, given obstacles such as ethical problems in treatment assignment, a practical problem of long-term adherence, and the current impossibility of double-blind treatment assignment [1]. Thus, for the alcohol-CVD question, we must scrutinize the available observational data, both retrospective and prospective, in an attempt to draw reasonable conclusions. In addition, some experimental data on the short term effect of alcohol on CVD risk factors are germane to the alcohol-CVD question.

## What is a Drink?

Drink standards vary, and are sized differently in, for example, North America, Europe, and Japan. In the U.K. a drink is 8 grams; in Denmark, 12 grams; in Canada, 13.75 grams; in the U.S.A. and Portugal, 14 grams; in Hungary, 17 grams; and in Japan, 18.75 grams.

In the U.S.A., reports variously refer to drinks per day, mls per day, or grams per day. The standard convention for drink size is 12 ounces of beer, 4 ½ ounces of wine, 1 ½ ounces of spirits, and 1 ounce of liqueur. The equivalent is mls of pure ethanol is 16 mls for a beer, 13 mls of a glass of wine, 18 mls for a mixed drink, and 11 mls for a liqueur. A convenient average is ½ ounce or 15 mls of ethanol per drink. Since the specific gravity of ethanol (compared to water) is about .79, 15 ml. of ethanol is about 12 grams. Clearly, some persons' drinks contain smaller amounts, and, more commonly, many persons' drinks contain larger amounts.

R. Paoletti et al. (eds.), Moderate Alcohol Consumption and Cardiovascular Disease, 23–36.

## The Effect of Alcohol on CVD Risk Factors

BLOOD PRESSURE

The literature is fairly congruent on the association of alcohol consumption with blood pressure; the greater the alcohol consumption, the greater the systolic and diastolic blood pressure [2,3] and rates of hypertension maybe double at higher levels of consumption [2]. However, many studies suggest a threshold effect, where there is little if any increase in blood pressure until drinking exceeds two drinks per day [3].

LIPIDS AND LIPOPROTEINS

One of the most consistent observations in previous studies has been the association of alcohol intake with increased high density lipoprotein cholesterol (HDL-C) [4]. This effect has been reported for both the major HDL-C subfractions, $HDL_2$-C and $HDL_3$-C [5], and for apolipoproteins A-I and AII [6]. The association shows a dose-response effect. A recent meta-analysis of alcohol and HDL-C in experimental studies showed that for 30 gm of ethanol, HDL-C increased 4.0 mg/dl, and apo AI increased 8.8 mg/dl [7].

Low density lipoprotein cholesterol (LDL-C) has been reported to be reduced with ethanol intake in some studies [8], but in one study this effect was present in women but not in men [9]. Experimental data are insufficient to estimate an average effect [7]. The results for triglycerides at moderate doses of alcohol have been inconsistent and variable. The above meta-analysis reported a small but significant 5.7 mg/dl increase in triglycerides per 30 gm of ethanol [7]. However, this association was not observed in women.

THROMBOTIC AND FIBRINOLYTIC FACTORS

*Thrombotic factors.* Significant reductions in fibrinogen [10] and measures of platelet aggregation [11] have been reported in several studies. Limited experimental data are available, and the methodology varies widely for platelet aggregation. For fibrinogen, the experimental data suggest a 7.5 mg/dl decrease for 30 gm of ethanol, but the 95% confidence interval included no change, perhaps due to the small number of studies [7]. Limited experimental data also suggest some reduction in Von-Willebrand factor and factor VII but sufficient data were not available to calculate a weighted average [7].

*Fibrinolytic factors.* Plasminogen and tissue type plasminogen activator (t-PA) have been reported to be higher in drinkers [12], but plasminogen activator inhibitor 1 (PAI-1) appears to be higher as well [13]. Lipoprotein (a), or lp(a), which may be involved in the fibrinolytic cascade, has been reported to be lower in drinkers [14]. Meta-analysis of the available experimental data for plasminogen, t-PA and lp(a) show findings in the above directions, but perhaps again because of a limited number of observations, the data were significant only for plasminogen [7].

INSULIN RESISTANCE

Both fasting and post-challenge insulin have been reported to be associated with alcohol intake [15,16] and similar findings have also been reported for post-challenge glucose [17,18]. Current experimental data on alcohol and insulin/glucose are insufficient to estimate an average effect [7]

## Alcohol and CVD Outcomes

Case-control and prospective studies are quite consistent in finding reduced coronary heart disease (CHD) in light to moderate drinkers. Figure 1, adapted from Marmot, shows that in men and women in prospective studies in diverse populations, moderate drinking is associated with a significant reduction in the risk of coronary events [19]. However, at heavier levels of drinking, the risk of all CVD actually tends to increase, producing a U-shaped relationship. Figure 2 illustrates this association in the Lipid Research Clinics Follow-up Study, separately for men and women [4]. Also, in some studies the risk of CHD increases at higher levels of alcohol consumption as well [4].

Several additional studies have now reported results for the other two major clinical manifestations of atherosclerotic CVD, stroke and peripheral arterial disease (PAD). Atherothrombotic stroke also shows an inverse relationship with alcohol for moderate consumption, although the U-shape curve with excess risk at higher levels of alcohol is much steeper than for CHD [20]. Hemorrhagic stroke shows a different relationship, with rates essentially increasing linearly with alcohol consumption [20]. PAD, like CHD and atherothrombotic stroke, shows a reduced risk with light-to-moderate alcohol intake [21]. Thus, the protective effect of alcohol in light to moderate amounts is specific for and limited to atherosclerotic CVD.

In terms of nonatherosclerotic CVD, alcohol at higher doses can elevate blood pressure [2,3], produce arrhythmias [22], and cause left ventricular hypertrophy and cardiomyopathy [23].

A concern has been raised that the usual reference group in studies of alcohol and CVD, nondrinkers, could result in bias if there were significant numbers of ex-drinkers who had quit because of CV conditions prior to baseline [24]. This issue has now been explored thoroughly in multiple cohorts by analyses excluding all participants with any history of CVD, and after these exclusions results continue to show a protective effect of alcohol for CVD [25]. In addition, never drinkers, where selective migration for ill health cannot, by definition, have occurred, have a higher risk of CHD than light to moderate drinkers [25]. Finally, it is interesting to note that due to misclassification any migration occurring after baseline would tend to obscure a true protective effect of alcohol [25].

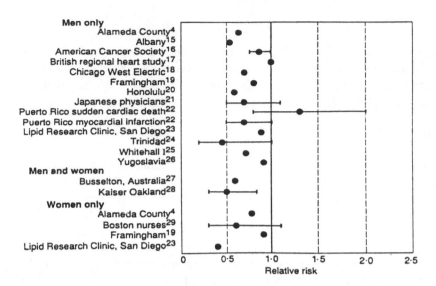

Figure 1. Relative risk of CHD in moderate versus nondrinkers, and 95% confidence interval (where available). Adapted from Marmot 1991 [19].

## Statistical Modeling of Potential Pathways for the Alcohol Effect

Although not experimental, prospective studies can help us explain the potential pathways for effects of alcohol on CVD, both beneficial and harmful. Such studies at baseline typically measure alcohol consumption along with a number of CVD risk factors which could be altered by ethanol and thus potential mediators of any alcohol effect on CVD events. Potential mediators include HDL-C, LDL-C, and systolic blood pressure (SBP). In two separate populations, we used multivariate models with CHD or CVD as the outcome variable, alcohol as the predictor variable, and HDL-C, LDL-C, and SBP as potential mediator variables. Traditional epidemiologic teaching has been to not include variables in multivariate models which might be intermediate variables in a causal chain between the predictor variable and the outcome variable, since the residual coefficient for the predictor variable would be diluted. However, we reasoned that by including and excluding such variables in alternate models we could determine both the direction and magnitude of any pathway effect of alcohol through such variables. Two papers were published in 1987 from the Lipid Research Clinic (LRC) Follow-up Study. The first showed that a 20 ml intake of ethanol per day was correlated with a reduced the risk of CVD death in men of about 20% [4]. Addition of HDL-C to the model reduced the apparent benefit of alcohol to 9%, a 55% change in the relative risk estimate, suggesting about 55% of the protective effect of alcohol was mediated by increased HDL-C. Addition of LDL-C to the model did not change the relative risk and thus indicated no mediation by LDL-C in this study.

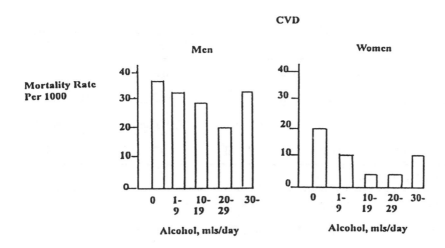

Figure 2. Age-adjusted mortality rates for men and women for CVD mortality by alcohol consumption category. Adapted from Criqui 1987 [4].

A second paper used similar analyses to evaluate a potential harmful effect of alcohol through a pathway of increased blood pressure [26] Addition of SBP to separate models for CHD and CVD death in men and CVD death in women increased the apparent alcohol benefit, indicating a harmful effect of alcohol through elevated SBP.

A paper in 1992 used similar methodology in the Honolulu Heart Study [27]. Comparable results were obtained. HDL-C appeared to explain about 47% of the benefit for alcohol. This study also showed a harmful effect of alcohol through increased SBP. Unlike the LRC study, this study showed a modest beneficial effect of alcohol through decreased LDL-C.

Table I summarizes findings from these two studies and similar analyses in two other epidemiologic studies [4,26-29]. Despite differences in study design, endpoints, and study size, the findings were remarkably similar. However, such analyses were observational and do not by themselves prove causality, despite their reproducibility.

What variables might mediate the "other half" of alcohol's protection? As noted earlier, salutary effects on thrombotic and fibrinolytic factors, as well as insulin resistance, have been described. The studies noted above did not have measurements on these factors at baseline and thus could not evaluate these potential pathways.

Table 1. Alcohol, HDL, and CHD/CVD in Four Epidemiological Studies*

|  | LRC Study | Honolulu Study | MRFIT Study | Boston Area Study |
|---|---|---|---|---|
| Study type | Cohort | Cohort | Cohort | Case-control |
| Baseline status | No CHD | No CVD | No CHD | MI/Controls |
| Endpoints | CVD death | Total CHD | CHD death | Nonfatal MI |
| Events/subjects | 130/4105 | 124/1768 | 190/1688 | 340/680 |
| Relative risk for alcohol |  |  |  |  |
| Alcohol | 0.80 | 0.83 | 0.89 | 0.60 |
| +HDL | 0.91 | 0.91 | 0.94 | 0.84 |
| % Δ in alcohol coeff. | 55% | 47% | 45% | 60% |

* Adapted from Criqui 1987 [4], Langer 1992 [27], Suh 1992 [28], and Graziano 1993 [29].

**Alcohol Effects in Specific Subgroups**

YOUNGER VERSUS OLDER

Intuitively, little benefit can be present in persons at very low risk of the one condition for which alcohol may have a benefit, atherosclerotic CVD. Klatsky et al. confirmed no benefit for alcohol in anyone under age 60 in a California HMO [30]. Fuchs et al. showed for women less than age 50 no mortality benefit in moderate drinkers, and a suggested hazard [31]. Thus, for younger individuals overall harm appeared to exceed benefit, while for older light to moderate drinkers, the risk ratio was reversed.

WOMEN VERSUS MEN

On average women have less total body water then men, and also metabolize ethanol differently, resulting in higher blood ethanol for a given intake [32]. In addition, alcohol appears to increase the risk of breast cancer, which is primarily a disease of women [33]. Thus, the harmful effects of alcohol are overall greater in women than men.

Low versus High Risk of CVD

Persons at higher risk of CVD should benefit more than persons at lower risk. In men, this supposition was confirmed in the British Regional Heart Study, where broad exclusions for CVD risk in men at baseline produced a group of men with few CVD events during follow-up and a predictable nonassociation with alcohol intake [34]. In women, Fuchs et al. showed an actual hazard for mortality of moderate alcohol intake in women free of CVD risk factors, while women with one or more CVD risk factors showed a significant benefit with light to moderate intake [31].

Primary versus Secondary Prevention

Most studies to date have been conducted on persons without known CVD at baseline (primary prevention). A recent report from the Physicians Health Study evaluated 5,358 men with a prior myocardial infarction (MI) (secondary prevention) [35]. This study showed a relative risk reduction similar to primary prevention studies, which translates to a much larger absolute risk reduction, since post-MI patients are at much higher risk than patients without CVD, and 77% of all deaths in this MI cohort were from CVD. Only 3.6% of this post-MI cohort drank two or more drinks per day, so the potential hazards of heavier drinking post-MI could not be evaluated [36].

Diabetes versus No Diabetes

Like post-MI patients, diabetes patients with or without a history of MI have an increased risk of CVD death [37]. A recent study evaluated the effect of alcohol consumption in 983 men and women with adult-onset diabetes [38]. As in the primary prevention study above, the risks of heavy drinking could not be estimated, due to only 3.8% of the population drinking more than two drinks per day. For light to moderate drinkers, the relative risk of CHD mortality was strikingly reduced, and this reduction was greater in both absolute and relative risk than in primary prevention studies. This finding raises the possibility of an effect of alcohol on insulin resistance in these patients. However, alcohol can both induce and mask severe hypoglycemia, and heavier alcohol intake can worsen diabetic neuropathy and actually exacerbate insulin resistance [39].

**Ecologic Studies and the French Paradox**

The studies discussed so far in this chapter have included retrospective case-control studies, prospective studies of defined cohorts, and short-term experimental studies of alcohol effects on potential mediating variables. In ecologic studies the units of analysis are large groups, typically an entire country. In such studies, for example, Food and Agriculture Organization (FAO) of the United Nations food disappearance data or other national data on diet can be used as independent variables, and World Health Organization (WHO) data on mortality as dependent variables. Such ecologic studies have shown that France has a low rate of CHD death, despite a relatively high intake of fat typical of Western diets; thus, "the French Paradox" [40-43]. Such study designs have the advantage of not having selective participation–essentially everyone is included. However, they have a disadvantage of not linking at an individual level exposure and outcome. Cultural variables across populations can occasionally result in an "ecological fallacy" where the association between an exposure and outcome at the level of the individual differs fom the association observed at the population level. However, for most exposures such a fallacy does not exist [44]. Table 2 below shows data from an ecologic study, with significant or borderline associations underlined [43]. For CHD mortality in 1980 and 1988, among the six dietary items shown, the only significant or suggestive multivariate associations were a positive association for animal fat, and inverse associations for wine ethanol and fruit. For total mortality however, wine ethanol was not protective, and beer ethanol showed a positive association. Only fruit remained protective for total mortality, underscoring the lack of benefit of alcohol for total mortality in populations.

Table 2. Multivariate Analysis of Dietary Items and CHD and Total Mortality, Men and Women Aged 35-74, 1980 and 1988*

|  | CHD Mortality | | | | Total Mortality | | | |
|  | 1980 | | 1988 | | 1980 | | 1988 | |
|  | Coeff | p value | Coeff | p value | Coeff | p value | Coeff | p value |
|---|---|---|---|---|---|---|---|---|
| Wine ethanol | INV | <.01 | INV | .12 | POS | NS | INV | NS |
| Beer ethanol | INV | NS | POS | NS | POS | .01 | POS | .05 |
| Spirits ethanol | INV | NS | INV | NS | INV | NS | POS | NS |
| Animal fat, % kcal | POS | .14 | POS | NS | INV | NS | INV | NS |
| Vegetables, % kcal | POS | NS | INV | NS | INV | NS | INV | NS |
| Fruit, %kcal | INV | .08 | INV | .06 | INV | .03 | INV | .05 |

*Adapted from Criqui et al. 1994 [43].

## Alcohol and Nonatherosclerotic Outcomes

Table 3 shows the association between alcohol at three levels of intake, with abstinence as the reference group, and various atherosclerotic and nonatherosclerotic outcomes [45]. For atherosclerotic outcomes, i.e. ischemic heart disease and most strokes, responsible drinking provided benefit. However, the relative risks for even responsible drinking were elevated for oropharyngeal, esophageal, liver, laryngeal, and female breast cancer, as well as liver cirrhosis. Hazardous and harmful drinking were associated with sharply increased risks for most outcomes.

Table 3. Pooled Estimates of Relative Risk for Neoplastic, Cardiovascular and Alimentary Diseases with Usual Alcohol Intakes, Classified by NHMRC Categories*

| | | Drinking pattern (drinks per day) | | | |
| | Studies in | Abstinence | Responsible | Hazardous | Harmful |
| Disease | meta-analysis | (0) | (>0-2.9) | (3-4.9) | (5+) |
|---|---|---|---|---|---|
| Oropharyngeal cancer | 4 | 1.00 | 1.45 | 1.85 | 5.39 |
| Oesophageal cancer | 7 | 1.00 | 1.80 | 2.37 | 4.26 |
| Liver cancer | 5 | 1.00 | 1.45 | 3.03 | 3.60 |
| Laryngeal cancer | 4 | 1.00 | 1.83 | 3.90 | 4.93 |
| Female breast cancer | 26 | 1.00 | 1.09 | 1.31 | 1.68 |
| Hypertension | 11 | | | | |
| men | | 1.00 | 1.02‡ | 1.43 | 2.05 |
| women | | 1.00 | 0.85 | 1.27 | 1.79 |
| Ischemic heart disease | 25 | 1.00 | 0.82 | 0.84 | 0.88 |
| Stroke | 21 | | | | |
| men | | 1.00 | 0.60 | 0.92‡ | 1.79 |
| women | | 1.00 | 0.58 | 0.48 | 7.96 |
| Liver cirrhosis | 7 | 1.00 | 1.26 | 9.54† | 9.54† |
| Cholelithiasis | 8 | 1.00 | 0.82 | 0.68 | 0.50 |

†, Combined; ‡, p = NS
*Adapted from Holman 1996 [45]

## Alcohol and Overall Risk

Figure 3 shows the association between alcohol intake and mortality in 276,802 men aged 40-49 in an American Cancer Society Prospective Study [46]. All-cause mortality was evaluated, as well as cause-specific mortality from CHD, stroke, cancer, and accidents and violence. These results are quite representative of epidemiologic studies overall. There was a benefit for both CHD and stroke, but this benefit was maximal at a single drink per day. Above one drink a day, the CHD benefit plateaued and the risk of stroke, as well as cancer and accidents and violence, increased, leading to an increase in total mortality at three or more drinks per day.

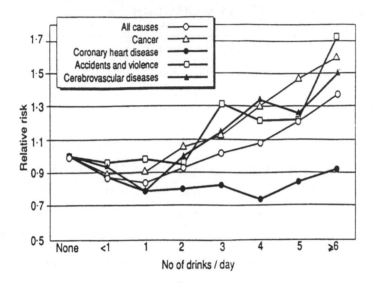

Figure 3. Relative risk of cause-specific and all-cause mortality in men by alcohol consumption category. Adapted from Bofetta 1990 [46].

As noted earlier, the mortality curves differ for men and women. Figure 4 is taken from a meta-analysis of 14 studies on the association of drinking and all-cause mortality [45]. Note the earlier upswing in the curve for women. These results illustrate that the daily limit for drinking in men should be around two, and in women around one.

The data shown so far in this chapter typically refer to age-adjusted morbidity or mortality. However, a fatal event at an early age produces many more potential years of life lost (PYLL) than a fatal event late in life. In fact, in women, CHD only ranks third as a cause of PYLL before age 75 [47]. Breast cancer is first, and motor vehicle crashes are second. Motor vehicle crashes are closely linked to alcohol consumption, and there is an association of alcohol with breast cancer. CHD does rank first in men as a cause of PYLL, but motor vehicle crashes are a closed second [47]. Thus, the overall harmful effects of alcohol are greater than can be appreciated in epidemiologic studies of largely middle-aged, responsible volunteers.

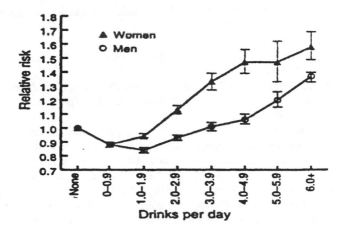

Figure 4. Relative risk of all-cause mortality in men and women by alcohol consumption category, a pooled analysis of 14 studies. Adapted from Holman 1996 [45].

## Should We Recommend Alcohol for Cardioprotection?

Skog has shown in a study across numerous populations that the percentage of a population drinking more than twice the mean is surprisingly constant, about 10-15%, irrespective of whether the mean consumption in 4 liters/year or 40 liters/year [48]. Interestingly, this 10-15% group consumes more than half the alcohol in most populations, indicating the dependence of alcohol sales on heavier drinking. Similarly, Rose has shown in the Intersalt Study that the correlation between mean population consumption of alcohol and heavy drinking is 0.97 [49]. The implications of these findings seem clear. Despite large cultural differences, the extent of ethanol abuse in a population is a direct function of mean consumption, and advocacy of drinking for health benefits will lead to increased consumption and harm to overall health.

There are selected situations where persons at higher risk of CVD with responsible drinking habits should discuss their alcohol intake with their physician. However, any more general recommendation is tantamount to recommending alcohol as a pharmaceutical for cardioprotection. If alcohol were a new unapproved pharmaceutical under regulatory review, phase I clinical trials in humans would reveal a dose-related suppression of cognition and coordination in all subjects, and developing dependency in about 10% of trial subjects. Irrespective of any potential benefits for CVD, such a drug would not be licensed because of the inherently high risk to benefit ratio [50].

## References

1.      Renaud S, Criqui MH, Farchi G, Veenstra J. Alcohol drinking and coronary heart disease.

In: Verschuren PM, editor. Health issues related to alcohol consumption. Washington: ILSI Press, 1993: 81-123.

2.      Klatsky AL, Friedman GD, Siegelaub AB, Gerard MJ. Alcohol consumption and blood pressure. Kaiser-Permanente Multiphasic Health Examination data. N Engl J Med 1977;296:1194-200.

3.      Criqui MH, Wallace RB, Mishkel M, Barrett-Connor E, Heiss G. Alcohol consumption and blood pressure. The Lipid Research Clinics Prevalence Study. Hypertension 1981;3:557-65.

4.      Criqui MH, Cowan LD, Tyroler HA, et al. Lipoproteins as mediators for the effects of alcohol consumption and cigarette smoking on cardiovascular mortality. Results from the Lipid Research Clinics Follow-up Study. Am J Epidemiol 1987;126:629-37.

5.      Haffner SM, Applebaum-Bowden D, Wahl PW, et al. Epidemiological correlates of high density lipoprotein subfractions, apolipoproteins A-I, A-II, and D, and lecithin cholesterol acyltransferase. Effects of smoking, alcohol, and adiposity. Arteriosclerosis1985;169-77.

6.      Camargo CA Jr, Williams PT, Vranizan KM, Albers JJ, Wood PD. The effect of moderate alcohol intake on serum apolipoproteins A-I and A-II. A controlled study. JAMA 1985; 17;253:2854-57.

7.      Rimm EB, Williams P, Forsher K, Criqui M, Stampfer MJ. Moderate alcohol intake and lower risk of coronary heart disease: Meta-analysis of effects on lipids and haemostatic factors. BMJ 1999;319:1523-28.

8.      Castelli WP, Doyle JT, Gordon T, et al. Alcohol and blood lipids. The cooperative lipoprotein phenotyping study. Lancet 1977;2:153-55.

9.      Criqui MH, Cowan LD, Heiss G, Haskell WL, Laskarzewski PM, Chambless LE. Frequency and clustering of non-lipid coronary risk factors in dyslipoproteinemia. The Lipid Research Clinics Program Prevalence Study. Circulation 1986;73 (Suppl 1):1-40-50.

10.     Meade TW, Chakrabarti R, Haines AP, North WR, Stirling Y. Characteristics affecting fibrinolytic activity and plasma fibrinogen concentrations. Br Med J 1979;1:153-56.

11.     Renaud SC, Beswick AD, Fehily AM, Sharp DS, Elwood PC. Alcohol and platelet aggregation: The Caerphilly Prospective Heart Disease Study. Am J Clin Nutr1992;1012-17.

12.     Ridker PM, Vaughan DE, Stampfer MJ, Glynn RJ, Hennekens CH. Association of moderate alcohol consumption and plasma concentration of endogenous tissue-type plasminogen activator. JAMA 1994;272:929-33

13.     Yarnell JW, Sweetnam PM, Rumley A, Lowe GD. Lifestyle and hemostatic risk factors for ischemic heart disease: The Caerphilly Study. Arterioscler Thromb Vasc Biol 2000;20:271-79.

14.     Valimaki M, Laitinen K, Ylikahri R, et al. The effect of moderate alcohol intake on serum apolipoprotein A-I-containing lipoproteins and lipoprotein (a). Metabolism 1991;40:1168-72

15.     Razay G, Heaton KW, Bolton CH, Hughes AO. Alcohol consumption and its relation to cardiovascular risk factors in British women. BMJ 1992;304:80-83.

16.     Kiechl S, Willeit J, Poewe W, et al. Insulin sensitivity and regular alcohol consumption: Large, prospective, cross sectional population study. BMJ 1996;313: 1040-44.

17.     Facchini, F; Chen, YD; Reaven, GM. Light-to-moderate alcohol intake associated with enhanced insulin sensitivity. Diabetes Care 1994; 17:115-19.

18.     Mayer EJ, Newman B, Quesenberry CP Jr, Friedman GD, Selby JV. Alcohol consumption

and insulin concentrations. Role of insulin in associations of intake with high-density lipoprotein cholesterol and triglycerides. Circulation 1993;88:2190-97.

19. Marmot M, Brunner E. Alcohol and cardiovascular disease: The status of the U shaped curve. BMJ 1991;303:565-68.

20. Kagan A, Yano K, Rhoads GG, McGee DL. Alcohol and cardiovascular disease: The Hawaiian experience. Circulation 1981;64:27-31.

21. Camargo CA Jr, Stampfer MJ, Glynn RJ, et al. Prospective study of moderate alcohol consumption and risk of peripheral arterial disease in US male physicians. Circulation 1997;95:577-80.

22. Ettinger PO, Wu CF, De La Cruz C Jr, Weisse AB, Ahmed SS, Regan TJ. Arrhythmias and the "holiday heart": Alcohol-associated cardiac rhythm disorders. Am Heart J 1978;95:555-62.

23. Urbano-Marquez A, Estruch R, Navarro-Lopez F, Grau JM, Mont L, Rubin E. The effects of alcoholism on skeletal and cardiac muscle. N Engl J Med 1989;320:409-15.

24. Shaper AG. Alcohol and mortality: A review of prospective studies. Br J Addict 1990; 85:837-47.

25. Criqui MH. The reduction of coronary heart disease with light to moderate alcohol consumption: effect or artifact? Br J Addict 1990;85:854-57.

26. Criqui MH. Alcohol and hypertension: New insights from population studies. European Heart Journal 1987;8 (Supplement B):19-26.

27. Langer RD, Criqui MH, Reed DM. Lipoproteins and blood pressure as biological pathways for effect of moderate alcohol consumption on coronary heart disease. Circulation 1992;85:910-15.

28. Suh I, Shaten BJ, Cutler JA, Kuller LH. Alcohol use and mortality from coronary heart disease: The role of high- lipoprotein cholesterol. The Multiple Risk Factor Intervention Trial Research Group. Ann Intern Med 1992;116:881-87.

29. Gaziano JM, Buring JE, Breslow JL, et al. Moderate alcohol intake, increased levels of high-density lipoprotein and its subfractions, and decreased risk of myocardial infarction. N Engl J Med 1993;16;329:1829-34.

30. Klatsky AL, Armstrong MA, Friedman GD. Alcohol and mortality. Ann Intern Med 1992;117:646-54.

31. Fuchs CS, Stampfer MJ, Colditz GA, et al. Alcohol consumption and mortality among women. N Engl J Med 1995;332:1245-50.

32. Dufour MC. Gender and race/ethnic differences in cardiovascular effects of alcohol. In: Sakhari S, Wassef M, editors. Alcohol and the cardiovascular system. NIAAA Research Monograph No. 31, 1996: 105-15.

33. Longnecker MP, Berlin JA, Orza MJ, Chalmers TC. A meta-analysis of alcohol consumption in relation to risk of breast cancer. JAMA 1988;260:652-56.

34. Shaper AG, Wannamethee G, Walker M. Alcohol and mortality in British men: Explaining the U-shaped curve. Lancet 1988;2:1267-73.

35. Muntwyler J, Hennekens CH, Buring JE, Gaziano JM. Mortality and light to moderate alcohol consumption after myocardial infarction. Lancet 1998;352:1882-85.

36. Criqui MH. Alcohol in the myocardial infarction patient. Lancet 1998;352:1873.

37. Haffner SM, Lehto S, Ronnemaa T, Pyorala K, Laakso M. Mortality from coronary heart disease in subjects with type 2 diabetes and nondiabetic subjects with and without prior myocardial infarction. N Engl J Med 1998;339:229-34.

38.     Valmadrid CT, Klein R, Moss SE, Klein BE, Cruickshanks KJ. Alcohol intake and the risk of coronary heart disease mortality in persons with older-onset diabetes mellitus. JAMA 1999;28:239-46.

39.     Criqui MH, Golomb BA. Should patients with diabetes drink to their health? JAMA 1999;282:279-80.

40.     St. Leger AS, Cochrane AL, Moore F. Factors associated with cardiac mortality in developed countries with particular reference to the consumption of wine. Lancet 1979;1:1017-20.

41.     Renaud S, de Lorgeril M. Wine, alcohol, platelets, and the French paradox for coronary heart disease. Lancet 1992;339:1523-6.

42.     Artaud-Wild SM, Connor SL, Sexton G, Connor WE. Differences in coronary mortality can be explained by differences in cholesterol and saturated fat intakes in 40 countries but not in France and Finland. A paradox. Circulation 1993;88:2771-79.

43.     Criqui MH, Ringel BL. Does diet or alcohol explain the French paradox? Lancet 1994; 344:1719-23.

44.     Criqui MH. Alcohol and coronary heart disease: A comparison of ecologic and non-ecologic studies: In: Gotto AM Jr, Lenfant C, Paoletti R, Catapano AL, Jackson AS, editors. Multiple risk factors in cardiovascular disease: Strategies of prevention of coronary heart disease, cardiac failure and stroke. Dordrecht: Kluwer Academic Publishers, 1998: 297-302.

45.     Holman CD, English DR, Milne E, Winter MG. Meta-analysis of alcohol and all-cause mortality: A validation of NHMRC recommendations. Med J Australia 1996;164:141-45.

46.     Boffetta P, Garfinkel L. Alcohol drinking and mortality among men enrolled in an American Cancer Society prospective study. Epidemiology 1990;1:342-48.

47.     Wilkins K, Mark E. Potential years of life lost, Canada 1990. Chronic Dis Canada 1992;13:111-15.

48.     Skog OJ. The collectivity of drinking cultures: A theory of the distribution of alcohol consumption. Br J Addict 1985; 80:83-99.

49.     Rose G. Ancel Keys Lecture. Circulation 1991;84:1405-9.

50.     Criqui MH. Moderate drinking: Benefits and risks. In: Sakhari S, Wassef M, editors. Alcohol and the cardiovascular system. NIAAA Research Monograph No. 31, 1996: 117-12.

MODERATE ALCOHOL CONSUMPTION AND HIGH DENSITY LIPOPROTEINS


Christian Ehnholm and Matti Jauhiainen


## Introduction

Epidemiological studies have shown that there is an J-shaped association between alcohol intake and coronary heart disease (CHD) [1]. Lighter drinkers have the lowest mortality risk and the curve has a nadir at one or two drinks per day. All mechanisms underlying the protective role of moderate alcohol consumption are not known at present but one may be an increase in plasma high density lipoprotein (HDL), a well-established marker associated with a reduced risk for atherosclerosis and myocardial infarction [2]. The aim of this presentation is to provide a review on how moderate alcohol consumption may lead to increased plasma levels of HDL and to focus on cellular and molecular mechanisms underlying the beneficial effects of moderate drinking.

HDL are the smallest and most dense among plasma lipoproteins. They originate in liver and intestine. Human plasma HDL consists of several subpopulations of particles with distinct structure, composition, and function. This heterogeneity, which is the result of continuous remodelling of HDL by plasma factors, has important implications for the cardioprotective function of HDL [3]. Proteins involved in the regulation of the subclass distribution of HDL include, lecithin:cholesterol acyltransferase (LCAT), phospholipid transfer protein (PLTP), cholesterol ester transfer protein (CETP), lipoprotein lipase (LPL), and hepatic lipase (HL).

The two distinct plasma lipid transfer proteins, CETP and PLTP, can markedly alter the size distribution of plasma lipoprotein fractions by shuttling lipid components from one lipoprotein substrate to another. CETP promotes the exchange of neutral lipids, cholesteryl esters, and triglycerides between nonequilibrated lipoprotein pools, leading to net transfer of cholesteryl esters from HDL toward triglyceride-rich lipoproteins and to transfer of triglycerides in the opposite direction [4]. The subsequent hydrolysis of transferred triglycerides by LPL and HL leads to the formation of small LDL and HDL particles [5].

A method that has been used to investigate the effects of alcohol on these factors and their influence on HDL metabolism has been to study patients suffering from alcoholism, a pathophysiological state that has been shown to be associated with abnormalities in plasma CETP activity, HDL profile, and alterations in plasma PLTP activity. Thus, alcohol withdrawal provides a unique opportunity to study *in vivo* alterations

37

R. Paoletti et al. (eds.), Moderate Alcohol Consumption and Cardiovascular Disease, 37–45.
© 2000 Kluwer Academic Publishers and Fondazione Giovanni Lorenzini. Printed in the Netherlands.

in plasma lipid transfer activities and to analyze their effects in terms of plasma HDL distribution.

## The Effect of Alcohol on the Size Distribution of Plasma High Density Lipoproteins

In human plasma, five distinct HDL subpopulations have been identified using polyacrylamide gradient native gel electrophoresis: $HDL_{2b}$ (9.7-12.9 nm), $HDL_{2a}$ (8.8-9.7 nm), $HDL_{3a}$ (8.2-8.8 nm), $HDL_{3b}$ (7.8-8.2 nm), and $HDL_{3c}$ (7.2-7.8 nm). It has been shown that coronary artery disease is strongly associated with abnormalities in HDL particle size distribution [6]. Therefore these observations raised a considerable interest in identifying the factors that can induce alterations in the relative proportions of plasma $HDL_{2b}$, $HDL_{2a}$, $HDL_{3a}$, $HDL_{3b}$, and $HDL_{3c}$ subfractions *in vivo*.

Recently Lagrost et al. [7])reported on the HDL size distribution in alcoholic patients before and after alcohol withdrawal. They demonstrated that the relative proportions of the largest HDL particles (i.e. $HDL_{2b}$ and $HDL_{2a}$) were significantly reduced after abstinence while the relative abundance of $HDL_{3a}$ remain unchanged. This is in good agreement with previous data [8,9] where the characteristic decrease in plasma HDL cholesterol observed after alcohol withdrawal was accompanied by a shift of HDL particle size towards smaller particles. This is in line with several studies that have reported that alcohol intake is associated with an increase in HDL size. Recently it has been shown that the clearance rate of HDL is a function of HDL size, small particles being cleared more efficiently [10].

## The Effect of Alcohol on HDL Synthesis and Remodeling

It is now well established that plasma HDL do not constitute stable entities *in vivo* but are continuously modified in the blood stream through the action of specific factors, i.e. LCAT, CETP, PLTP, LPL, and HL. The participation of these proteins in HDL metabolism is schematically depicted in Figure 1.

The main protein constituents of HDL, apoA-I and apoA-II, are synthesized in liver and gut and are secreted into the circulation in the form of discoidal particles containing the apoprotein complexed with phospholipid and free cholesterol. Similar discoidal "nascent" HDL particles are also generated when redundant surface components are shed from chylomicrons (CM) and very low density lipoproteins (VLDL) during lipolysis. The discoidal HDL acquire free cholesterol from cell membranes and other lipoproteins. Free cholesterol is rapidly esterified by LCAT. The esterified cholesterol formed is highly hydrophobic and generates a core in the discoidal HDL particles which are converted into spherical HDL. Further esterification then increases HDL size. As the HDL particles increase in size they can acquire additional lipid-poor apoA-I [3]. LCAT may also promote fusion of spherical A-I HDL with discoidal A-II HDL particles and thereby result in the formation of A-I/A-II HDL.

Effect of alcohol on hepatic apoA-I biosynthesis has been followed in kinetic studies in healthy volunteers before and after a one-month period of alcohol use. It was shown that the biosynthetic rate of apoA-I was increased thus providing support for the increased levels of plasma HDL cholesterol. However, this study did not differentiate if the effect of ethanol is exerted in the hepatocytes, in the intestine, or both of them [11]. Increase in apoA-I synthesis was supported by findings from primary cultures of hepatocytes from ethanol-fed rats. These hepatocytes secreted more apoA-I than the control cells [12].

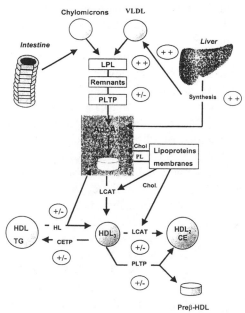

Figure 1. Participation of lipolytic enzymes and plasma lipid transfer proteins in HDL metabolism. In the circulation apoA-I, biosynthesized in the liver, accepts phospholipids and cholesterol from lipoproteins and cell membranes and forms nascent discoidal HDL particles. HDL discs are good substrates for LCAT and the discs are transformed to spherical HDL particles containing cholesterol ester core. Further reaction with LCAT transforms the $HDL_3$ to a larger $HDL_2$. The cholesterol esters formed can be transported with the aid of the CETP to LDL and VLDL in exchange with TG. This leads to HDL particles with increased TG content. The TG-enriched HDL are good substrates for HL and HL reduces the size of HDL accompanied with a release of lipid poor apoA-I. Small HDL particles, especially $HDL_3$, are preferential substrates for PLTP-mediated HDL conversion. This process leads to the formation of large, $HDL_2$-like fusion particles as well as small, lipid poor apoA-I containing preβ-HDL particles known to be the primary cholesterol acceptors from peripheral cells in the reverse cholesterol transport process. In addition, PLTP is also involved in the transfer of VLDL surface remnants, mainly phospholipids, to HDL during LPL-mediated lipolysis. Signs indicate the increasing (+) or decreasing (-) effect of alcohol on these processes.

## The Effect of Alcohol on LCAT

LCAT catalyzes the transfer of fatty acids from the sn-2 position of phosphatidylcholine (PC) to cholesterol, producing cholesterol ester and lyso-PC. The formation of the nonpolar cholesterol ester depletes the free cholesterol from the surface of HDL thus maintaining a free cholesterol concentration gradient and promoting the reverse cholesterol transport of cholesterol from peripheral tissues to liver [13]. HDL are the preferred substrates for LCAT, and apolipoprotein A-I (apoA-I), the major protein component of HDL, is the main activator of the enzyme. In human plasma, LCAT is responsible for the formation of the major portion of total cholesterol esters.

The effect of alcohol on LCAT activity has been studied in order to explain the mechanism whereby alcohol increases HDL levels. In a study by Nishiwaki et al. [14] after 3 weeks of abstinence, 12 men consumed 0.5 g/kg body weight of alcohol per day for 4 weeks and 13 abstaining men served as controls. This moderate alcohol intake did not affect plasma LCAT activity, and therefore LCAT was not considered to be a contributor to the HDL cholesterol elevation that followed alcohol intake. This result was in line with that reported by Albers et al. [15] and recently by Riemens et al. [16] who observed no differences in LCAT activity between alcohol users and nonusers. In addition to LCAT activity, Haffner et al. [17] observed no correlation between plasma LCAT protein mass and alcohol consumption. In one study the effect of moderate doses of alcoholic beverages on LCAT and HDL in postprandial state were studied [18]. Alcohol was consumed as beer, wine or spirits before and during dinner thus simulating social type of drinking. HDL triglycerides were elevated at 5 and 9 hours whereas HDL cholesterol was elevated at 13 hours postprandially. Plasma LCAT activity was slightly increased 9 hours after dinner and the increased activities were similar for all three alcoholic beverages. It can be concluded that moderate alcohol use has a very modest effect on the activity of plasma LCAT.

## The Effect of Alcohol on Lipid Transfer Proteins, CETP and PLTP

The two plasma lipid transfer proteins, CETP and PLTP, are important factors in the regulation of HDL levels and HDL metabolism. After cholesterol esterification by LCAT within the HDL fraction, CETP catalyzes the transfer of cholesteryl ester from HDL towards VLDL, IDL, and LDL in exchange for triglycerides. This leads to lowering of HDL cholesterol [19]. PLTP only transfers phospholipids between HDL and VLDL [20] and in a model system between liposomes and HDL [21]. It also transfers phospholipids between particles within the HDL fraction in a process which results in the conversion of HDL into larger and smaller particles. Recent studies suggest that the major *in vivo* functions of PLTP are (i) to facilitate the HDL remodelling to form large HDL fusion particles and small preβ-mobile apoA-I-phospholipid complexes capable of accepting cholesterol from peripheral cells [22,23] and (ii) to mediate transfer of phospholipids from VLDL remnants to HDL [24]. Therefore, PLTP appears to be a central regulator of plasma HDL. It controls the overall plasma HDL level and plays a pivotal role in the antiatherogenic reverse cholesterol transport process.

The effect of alcohol on plasma CETP and PLTP activities has been investigated both in moderate alcohol consumers and in alcohol-abusers. Between heavy and moderate alcohol use there is a clear difference in plasma CETP. Savolainen et al.[25] and recently Lagrost et al. [7] reported low CETP activity and high HDL cholesterol levels in alcoholic patients consuming more than 100 g of alcohol per day. Similar results were obtained in alcoholic women [9]. Hannuksela et al. [26] furthermore reported that also CETP mass was low in alcohol-abusers. After alcohol withdrawal, plasma CETP activity increased with a concomitant fall in HDL cholesterol levels.

In contrast to the results observed in alcoholic subjects, no effect of moderate alcohol intake on the plasma CETP activity could be demonstrated although a beneficial increase in HDL cholesterol levels was observed [14,16]. These contrasting findings may be due to differences in the duration and mode of alcohol intake, diet, the susceptibility of the study subjects to ingested alcohol, hepatotoxic effect of alcohol and the CETP assay methods. Since liver is an important biosynthetic site for circulatory CETP, the lower CETP activity in alcoholics may to some extent be due to ethanol-mediated liver injury. This aspect is supported by the finding that in alcohol abusers plasma CETP activity is negatively correlated with alanine aminotransferase (ALAT) levels [9].

The data on the effects of alcohol on plasma PLTP activity are analogous to those of CETP, i.e. moderate alcohol intake does not affect PLTP activity despite the increased HDL cholesterol levels [16]. In male alcohol abusers, however, the net mass transfer of phospholipids was four-fold higher as compared to controls, and PLTP activity increased by 33% [27]. This result is in good agreement with the report where PLTP activity was determined in 33 alcoholic patients entering a cessation program. Alcohol withdrawal was associated with a significant reduction in PLTP activity [7].

We have recently observed , based on PLTP mass measurement, that plasma PLTP activity and mass do not correlate and that plasma contains PLTP both in inactive and active form [28]. Therefore, it will be of great interest to investigate whether alcohol use will selectively affect either the inactive or the active PLTP pools.

The data so far published suggest that the high HDL cholesterol level associated with moderate alcohol consumption is unlikely to be caused by LCAT, CETP, or PLTP.

## The Effect of Alcohol on Lipolytic Enzymes

A number of studies have implicated the two heparin releasable endothelial lipases, LPL and HL, in regulating plasma HDL levels [29]. LPL plays a central role in lipoprotein metabolism, hydrolyzing both dietary and endogenous triglycerides transported in VLDL particles [30]. However, there is growing evidence that LPL is a multifunctional protein that, in addition to its lipolytic function, also can mediate the uptake and degradation of lipoproteins by cells [31].

HL is synthesized by hepatocytes and mainly localized to hepatic sinusoids. HL has both triglyceride hydrolase and phospholipase $A_1$ activity [32]. HL is important in the metabolism of intermediate-density lipoprotein (IDL) triglyceride as well as in the hydrolysis of HDL triglyceride and phospholipids. HL does not require an apoprotein activator for activity but apoproteins have a major influence on HL-mediated phospholipid and triacylglycerol hydrolysis of HDL [33]. Studies in transgenic animals have provided evidence that in addition to its catalytic activity HL can also act as a ligand to remove lipoproteins from plasma [34].

LPL can affect HDL metabolism in several ways. Current evidence indicates that one role LPL may play is to regulate HDL levels by hydrolyzing core triglycerides of VLDL and chylomicrons resulting in the transfer of redundant surface components such as phospholipid and cholesterol to nascent HDL which, following the action of LCAT, results in the formation of mature HDL particles [35]. This transfer of phospholipids between VLDL and HDL is stimulated by the phospholipid transfer protein (PLTP) [24].

In addition to its role in remnant metabolism, HL hydrolyzes both triglycerides and phospholipids in HDL. The plasma levels of HDL are inversely correlated to HL activity in postheparin plasma [29]. The hydrolysis of HDL lipids by HL results in the conversion of large boyuant $HDL_2$ to smaller and more dense $HDL_3$ particles. During this process as the volume of the HDL particle decreases, lipid-poor apoA-I is released [36]. This lipid-poor apoA-I is a preferred acceptor of cell-membrane cholesterol and plays an important role in reverse cholesterol transport. By causing interconversion of HDL HL not only influences the distribution of HDL subclasses but also affects HDL turnover. Thus the role of HL in HDL metabolism is of considerable importance as shown by the strong negative association between HL activity and plasma $HDL_2$ levels [37].

The influence of alcohol on the activities of the endothelial lipases depends on ethanol dose, acute versus chronic intake, species studied and degree of liver damage and consequently a wide range of responses has been reported for these two enzymes including no effect, depressed, and accentuated activity. It seems that acute intake of alcohol may have a transient inhibitory effect on LPL that returns to normal levels after 10 hours [38]. While prolonged consumption of alcohol seems to lead to an increase in LPL activity [39] this may be a compensatory response to accentuated hepatic VLDL synthesis. The concentration of HDL specifically $HDL_2$ in plasma appear to be controlled by the balance of LPL versus HL activity, with LPL enhancing $HDL_2$ formation and HL promoting its clearance from the circulation [8,38]. Thus an increase in LPL in conjunction with a smaller change in HL activity would result in an increase in HDL formation and maintain plasma triglyceride (VLDL) at normal levels. This intravascular HDL production along with enhanced *de novo* hepatic HDL synthesis would lead to higher plasma HDL levels.

## Conclusions

A strong positive relationship between alcohol consumption and HDL cholesterol level has been established in cross-sectional studies within populations. Social drinkers have mean HDL levels that may be higher than those of teetotalers by as much as 30%. It has been estimated that alcohol consumption accounts for at least 4 to 6% and possibly up to 10%

of the total variation of HDL cholesterol in Western industrialized populations. The smallest daily dose of alcohol, by which significant increases of HDL cholesterol or apoproteins are achieved, is about 30 to 40 g. The molecular mechanisms underlying the increase in plasma HDL are far from resolved. At present an increased hepatic synthesis of VLDL and nascent HDL in combination with changes in the activities of lipolytic enzymes seem to be the main metabolic alterations that can explain the HDL elevation.

## References

1.   Boffeta P, Garfinkel L. Alcohol drinking and mortality among men enrolled in an American Cancer Society prospective study. Epidemiology 1990;1:342-48.
2.   Gordon DJ, Rifkind BM. High density lipoprotein: The clinical implication of recent studies. NEJM 1998;321:1311-16.
3.   Rye K-A, Clay MA, Barter PJ. Remodeling of high density lipoproteins by plasma factors. Atherosclerosis 1999;145:227-38.
4.   Tall AR. Plasma lipid transfer proteins. Ann Rev Biochem 1995;64:235-57.
5.   Clay MA, Newnham HH, Forte TM, Barter PJ. Cholesteryl ester transfer protein and hepatic lipase activity promote shedding of apoA-I from HDL and subsequent formation of discoidal HDL. Biochim Biophys Acta 1992;1124:52-58.
6.   Cheung MC, Brown BG, Wolf AC, Albers JJ. Altered particle size distribution of apolipoprotein A-I containing lipoprotein in subjects with coronary artery disease. J Lipid Res 1991;32:383-94.
7.   Lagrost L, Athias A, Herbeth B, et al. Opposite effects of cholesteryl ester transfer protein and phospholipid transfer protein on the size distribution of plasma high density lipoproteins. Physiological relevance in alcoholic patients. J Biol Chem 1996;271:19058-65.
8.   Taskinen M-R, Välimäki M, Nikkilä EA, Kuusi T, Ehnholm C, Ylikahri R. High density lipoprotein subfractions and postheparin plasma lipases in alcoholic men before and after ethanol withdrawal. Metabolism 1982;31:1168-74.
9.   Välimäki M, Kahri J, Laitinen K, et al. High density lipoprotein subfractions, apolipoprotein A-I containing lipoproteins, lipoprotein (a), and cholesteryl ester transfer protein activity in alcoholic women before and after ethanol withdrawal. Eur J Clin Invest 1993;23:406-17.
10.  Lamarche B, Uffelman KD, Carpentier A, et al. Triglyceride enrichment of HDL enhances in vivo metabolic clearance of HDL apoA-I in healthy men. J Clin Invest 1999;103:1191-99.
11.  Malmendier CL, Delcroix C. Effect of alcohol intake on high- and low-density lipoprotein metabolism in healthy volunteers. Clin Chim Acta 1985;152:281-28.
12.  Lin RC, Lumeng L, Phelps VL. Serum high-density lipoprotein particles of alcohol-fed rats are deficient in apolipoprotein E. Hepatology 1989;9:307-13
13.  Fielding CJ, Fielding PE. Molecular physiology of reverse cholesterol transport. J Lipid Res 1995;36:211-28.
14.  Nishiwaki M, Ishikawa T, Ito T, et al. Effects of alcohol on lipoprotein lipase, hepatic lipase, cholesteryl ester transfer protein, and lecithin-cholesterol acyltransferase in high-density lipoprotein cholesterol elevation. Atherosclerosis 1994;111:99-109.

15.     Albers JJ, Bergelin RO, Adolphson JL, Wahl PW. Population-based reference values for lecithin-cholesterol acyltransferase (LCAT). Atherosclerosis 1982;43:369-74.
16.     Riemens SC, van Tol A, Hoogenberg K, et al. Higher high density lipoprotein cholesterol associated with moderate alcohol consumption is not related to altered plasma lecithin-cholesterol acyltransferase and lipid transfer protein activity levels. Clin Chim Acta 1997; 258:105-15.
17.     Haffner SM, Applebaum-Bowden D, Wahl PW, et al. Epidemiological correlates of high density lipoprotein subfractions, apolipoprotein A-I, A-II, and D, and lecithin cholesterol acyltransferase. Effects of smoking, alcohol, and adiposity. Arteriosclerosis 1985;5:169-76.
18.     Hendriks HFJ, Veenstra J, van Tol A, Groener JEM, Schaafsma G. Moderate doses of alcoholic beverages with dinner and postprandial high density lipoprotein composition. Alcohol and Alcoholism 1998;33:403-10.
19.     Tall AR, Breslow JL. Plasma high density lipoproteins and atherogenesis. In: Fuster V, Ross R, Topol EJ, editors. Atherosclerosis and coronary artery disease. Philadelphia: Lippincott-Raven Publishers, 1996:105-28.
20.     Tollefson JH, Ravnik S, Albers JJ. Isolation and characterization of a phospholipid transfer protein (LTP-II) from human plasma. J Lipid Res 1988;29:1593-1602
21.     Jauhiainen M, Ehnholm C. Role of the plasma phospholipid transfer protein in plasma lipid transport. In: Barter PJ, Rye K-A, editors. Plasma lipids and their role in disease. Amsterdam: Harwood Academic Publishers, 1999:285-97.
22.     Von Eckardstein A, Jauhiainen M, Huang Y et al. Phospholipid transfer protein mediated conversion of high density lipoproteins generates prebeta-1-HDL. Biochim Biophys Acta 1996;1301:255-62.
23.     Wolfbauer G, Albers JJ, Oram JF. Phospholipid transfer protein enhances removal of cellular cholesterol and phospholipids by high-density lipoprotein apolipoproteins. Biochim Biophys Acta 1999;1439:65-76.
24.     Jiang XC, Bruce C, Mar J et al. Targeted mutation of plasma phospholipid transfer protein gene markedly reduces high-density lipoprotein levels. J Clin Invest 1999;103:907-14.
25.     Savolainen MJ, Hannuksela M, Seppänen S, Kervinen K, Kesäniemi YA. Increased high-density lipoprotein cholesterol concentration in alcoholics is related to low cholesteryl ester transfer protein activity. Eur J Clin Invest 1990;20:593-99.
26.     Hannuksela M, Marcel YL, Kesäniemi A, Savolainen MJ. Reduction in the concentration and activity of plasma cholesteryl ester transfer protein by alcohol. J Lipid Res 1992;33: 737-44.
27.     Liinamaa MJ, Hannuksela ML, Kesäniemi YA, Savolainen MJ. Altered transfer of cholesteryl esters and phospholipids in plasma from alcohol abusers. Arterioscler Thromb Vasc Biol 1997;17:2940-47.
28.     Huuskonen J, Ekström M, Tahvanainen E, et al. Quantification of human plasma phospholipid transfer protein (PLTP): Relationship between PLTP mass and phospholipid transfer activity. Atherosclerosis 2000, in press.
29.     Kuusi T, Ehnholm C, Viikari J, Harkonen R, Vartiainen E, Puska P, Taskinen, M-R. Postheparin plasma lipoprotein and hepatic lipase are determinants of hypo-and hyperalphalipoproteinemia, J Lipid Res 1989;30:1117-26.
30.     Olivecrona T, Bengtsson-Olivecrona G. Lipoprotein lipase and hepatic lipase. Curr Opin Lipidol 1993;4:187-96.

31.     Beisiegel U, Weber W, Bengtsson-Olivecrona G. Lipoprotein lipase enhances the binding of chylomicrons to low density lipoprotein receptor related protein. Proc Natl Acad Sci USA 1991;88:8342-46.
32.     Ehnholm C, Kuusi T. Preparation, characterization and measurement of hepatic lipase. Methods in Enzymology 1986;129:716-38.
33.     Hime NJ, Barter PJ, Rye K-A. The influence of apolipoprotein on the hepatic lipase-mediated hydrolysis of high density lipoprotein phospholipid and triacylglycerol. J Biol Chem 1999;273:27191-99.
34.     Dichek HL, Brecht W, Fan J, et al. Overexpression of hepatic lipase in transgenic mice decreases apolipoprotein B-containing and high density lipoproteins. Evidence that hepatic lipase acts as a ligand for lipoprotein uptake. J Biol Chem 1998;273, 1896-1903.
35.     Clay MA, Barter PJ. Formation of new HDL particles from lipid-free apolipoprotein A-I. J Lipid Res 1996;37:1722-32.
36.     Marques-Vidal P, Jauhiainen M, Metso J, Ehnholm C. Transformation of high density lipoprotein 2 particles by hepatic lipase and phospholipid transfer protein. Atherosclerosis. 1997;133:87-95.
37.     Guerra R, Wang J, Grundy SM and Cohen JC. A hepatic lipase (LIPC) allele associated with high plasma concentrations of high density lipoprotein cholesterol. Proc Natl Acad Sci USA 1997; 94:4532-37.
38.     Nikkilä EA. HDL in relation to the metabolism of triglyceride rich lipoproteins. In: Miller NE, Miller GJ, editors. Clinical and metabolic aspects of high density lipoproteins, New York: Elsevier, 1984:215-24.
39.     Taskinen M-R, Välimäki M, Nikkilä EA, Kuusi T, Ylikahri R. Sequence of alcohol-induced initial changes in plasma lipoproteins (VLDL and HDL) and lipolytic enzymes in humans. Metabolism 1985;34:112-19.

ACUTE EFFECTS OF ALCOHOL ON THE TURNOVER OF VERY LOW DENSITY LIPOPROTEIN (VLDL) APOLIPOPROTEIN B-100 IN NORMOLIPIDEMIC SUBJECTS

Henry J. Pownall, Diane H. Bick, Kay T. Kimball, Danièle Zoch, and Christie M. Ballantyne

Consumption of alcohol, prescribed by physicians of ancient Mesopotamia and Egypt and described as native to several hundred preliterate societies, would seem to be as old as humankind [1]. Today alcohol is consumed in most countries; traditional patterns of drinking vary from occasional, celebratory use to alcohol's role as part of the usual diet [2]. In the United States, 63% of men and 45% of women reported consuming alcohol during the past year in the 1992 National Health Interview Surveys [3], and also in 1992, according to the National Longitudinal Alcohol Epidemiologic Survey, approximately 14 million (or 7.4% of) U.S. adults met standard diagnostic criteria for alcohol abuse or alcohol dependence [4]. The Janus-like character of alcohol consumption is underscored in its J-shaped relation to total mortality rate:lowest mortality occurs in those who consume one or two drinks per day, and total mortality rises rapidly with increasing number of drinks as they exceed three per day [5,6]. The well-demonstrated cardioprotective effect of moderate alcohol consumption plays a key role in that relation. A consistent 30-50% reduction in relative risk for coronary heart disease has been reported among moderate drinkers in disparate populations [6,7].

An increase in plasma concentrations of high-density lipoprotein (HDL) cholesterol has been suggested to mediate about half of the cardioprotective effect of alcohol [6-9]. However, alcohol elicits other lipid changes that may be mechanistically linked to the effect. For example, alcohol increases the total turnover and synthetic rates of very low density lipoprotein (VLDL) triglyceride (TG) [10] and acutely increases plasma TG concentration in normotriglyceridemic [11-16] but not hypertriglyceridemic [16] subjects. Moreover, the lipemic response to an acute alcohol load is markedly enhanced by dietary fat [17-20], an effect that has been attributed to the inhibition of lipolysis of intestinally derived lipoproteins [15,19]. That inhibitory effect could be specific to the intestinally derived lipoproteins, or it could be a general effect that would also include VLDL, which is hepatically derived. The present study was therefore conducted to determine whether alcohol given acutely inhibits VLDL turnover.

47

R. Paoletti et al. (eds.), Moderate Alcohol Consumption and Cardiovascular Disease, 47–52.
© 2000 Kluwer Academic Publishers and Fondazione Giovanni Lorenzini. Printed in the Netherlands.

## Methods

### SUBJECTS AND EXPERIMENTAL DESIGN

Subjects were healthy, nonalcoholic, normolipidemic adults (total cholesterol $\leq$ 200 mg/dL, HDL cholesterol > 35 mg/dL, TG < 200 mg/dL, and LDL cholesterol $\leq$ 130 mg/dL). The 8 men and 5 women ranged in age from 23 to 62 years; their mean plasma lipid concentrations $\pm$ SEM were total cholesterol 170.4 $\pm$ 5.8 mg/dL, HDL cholesterol 47.7 $\pm$ 2.3 mg/dL, TG 145.2 $\pm$ 10.9 mg/dL, and LDL cholesterol 93.8 $\pm$ 4.4 mg/dL. LDL cholesterol values were calculated by the Friedewald formula [21]; values of the other major lipid fractions were determined by enzymatic methods in the Lipid Laboratory of the Section of Atherosclerosis and Lipoprotein Research, Baylor College of Medicine. The protocol was approved by the Institutional Review Board of The Methodist Hospital and Baylor College of Medicine. After an overnight fast, subjects drank either 400 mL of water or 40 mL of alcohol in 360 mL of water; each subject underwent both tests. Subjects were injected with a bolus of [125I]-labeled autologous VLDL and blood samples (10 mL) were collected from a contralateral intravenous line kept open by a saline infusion. After the injection, subjects were allowed free access to water for the duration of the blood collection.

### RADIOIODINATION OF AUTOLOGOUS VLDL

VLDL was isolated from each patient by preparative ultracentrifugation and floated at a density of 1.004 g/mL. The VLDL was iodinated with [125I] by using the iodine monochloride method of Bilheimer et al. [22]. Unbound radioactive iodine was removed by extensive dialysis against 0.15 mmol/L NaCl and 0.26 mmol/L EDTA. The content of unbound radioactive iodine was below 1% as assessed by protein precipitation with 10% trichloracetic acid and 5% phosphotungstic acid. The extent of lipid labeling was less than 10% and was monitored by extracting the [125I]VLDL with 2:1 chloroform/methanol solvent. [125I]VLDL was then sterilized by filtration and the level of endotoxin screened by using the Limulus Amebocyte Lysate kit (Biowhittaker, Walkerville, MD). The injected VLDL contained 35-50 $\mu$Ci of radiolabel and 2.5-5 mg VLDL protein in a 1- to 2-mL injection volume.

### PLASMA DECAY OF [125I]VLDL

After injection of the [125I]VLDL, blood samples were collected at 15 and 30 minutes, then hourly from 1-12 hours. Aprotinin was added to a final concentration of 10 kallikrein inhibitory units (KIU) per mL of plasma and phenylmethylsulfonylfluoride (PMSF) to 1 mmol/L. The samples were then fractionated by spinning the plasma on a gradient, using a modification of the procedure of Lindgren et al. [23]. The density of 4 mL of plasma was adjusted to a density of 1.386 g/mL with NaBr in a Beckman SW40 centrifuge tube.

Layered on top of the plasma sample were 3.8 mL of $d = 1.063$ g/mL NaBr, 3.3 mL of 1.019 g/mL NaBr, and 0.8 mL of 1.006 g/mL NaBr. The tubes were then spun at 40,000 rpm for 22 hours at 20°C. The resulting gradients were fractionated into 0.3-mL fractions. Apo B-100 of the fractions was precipitated by using the isopropanol method of Egusa et al. [24]. Apo B-100 radioactivity was counted and protein was measured by using the BCA kit (Pierce, Rockford, IL). Decay of apo B-100–specific radioactivity from the VLDL fraction was fitted by using a nonlinear regression analysis to calculate a rate constant for the loss of radioactivity from VLDL. For comparison, all data are normalized to the same value at 1 hour.

STATISTICAL METHODS

Differences between decay constants following consumption of alcohol and water or water alone were tested by a one-sided Wilcoxon signed ranks test. The alternative hypothesis was that the rate of decay of VLDL [$^{125}$I] apo B-100 after an acute dose of alcohol would be significantly inhibited. The statistical analyses were performed using STATA Release 5.0 (Stata Corporation, College Station, TX, 1997).

**Results and Discussion**

Label disappearance at 15 minutes and from 0-12 hours is shown in Figure 1.The median rate constant for the disappearance of VLDL [$^{125}$I] apo B-100 was 0.17 h$^{-1}$ (range 0.06–0.46 h$^{-1}$) after the ingestion of alcohol and water, compared with 0.14 h$^{-1}$ (range 0.09–0.39 h$^{-1}$) after the ingestion of water alone, a statistically significant difference ($P = 0.044$). In addition, the observed heterogeneity in rate constants was greater after alcohol than water ingestion.

Among normolipidemic subjects, acute alcohol ingestion produces a transient increase in plasma TG [11-16]. Regular, moderate consumption of alcohol produces a TG increase that is more persistent [25-27]. In addition, alcohol enhances postprandial lipemia [17-20], by an unknown mechanism. Possible mechanisms are inhibition of hepatic or lipoprotein lipase, increased production of VLDL TG, or decreased clearance of TG-rich lipoprotein remnants. Acutely, alcohol decreases plasma concentrations of nonesterified fatty acids, an effect that could be due to decreased lipolysis in both tissue and the plasma compartment. In a turnover study using radiolabeled palmitate, it was suggested that alcohol decreases the influx of nonesterified fatty acids from adipose tissue to plasma [28]. Those findings are consistent with a study showing that alcohol inhibits the hydrolysis of intestinally derived lipoproteins [15], an effect that could be due to the inhibition of hepatic or lipoprotein lipase. Studies of the effects of alcohol on postheparin lipases, however, are not in total agreement. After acute alcohol intake postheparin lipolytic activity has been reported to decrease [29,30] or to remain unchanged [19,31]. As an alternative method, we measured the turnover of VLDL particles by following the clearance kinetics for VLDL [$^{125}$I] apoB-100.

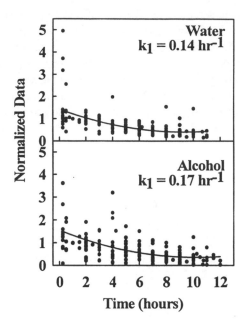

Figure 1. Turnover of VLDL [$^{125}$I]apolipoprotein B-100 in 12 normolipidemic subjects after ingestion of 400 mL water (top) or 40 mL alcohol in 360 mL water (bottom). Curves were fitted to a first-order decay of the mean specific activities at each time point.

The inhibition of hydrolysis by alcohol shown for intestinally derived lipoproteins does not appear to occur with lipoproteins of hepatic origin. In fact, our data showed an increase rather than a decrease in VLDL [$^{125}$I]apo B-100 turnover after acute alcohol ingestion. Although the difference between alcohol and water was statistically significant, the increased turnover of apo B-100 by alcohol relative to water was relatively small (+14%). This is in stark contrast to the effects of alcohol on chylomicron hydrolysis, where there is a greater than 90% reduction in the release of fatty acids. There are several possible explanations for the different results for TG-rich lipoproteins of hepatic and intestinal origin. One possibility is that VLDL particles are more susceptible to hydrolysis than chylomicrons. Most data, however, show that the opposite is true: chylomicron turnover occurs on a time scale of minutes, whereas VLDL turnover is on a time scale of hours. Another possibility is that an inhibitor is released into or activated within the plasma compartment only when fat and alcohol are consumed together. If that model is correct, tests of VLDL turnover similar to the present study could be conducted following simultaneous ingestion of fat and alcohol.

In spite of much work on the topic, the mechanism by which alcohol elicits its cardioprotective effect is not established. Because most people consume alcohol with food, elucidating the interaction of dietary fat and alcohol is central to understanding the mechanism. Studies of the effects of regular consumption of moderate amounts of alcohol on factors such as postprandial lipemia and plasma homocysteine concentration are needed to guide the design of cell studies to better define the cardioprotective mechanism.

## Acknowledgment

This work was supported by a grant-in-aid from the Washington Technical Information Group, Inc, Washington, DC.

## References

1.  Alcohol consumption. Encyclopædia Britannica Online. <http://www.eb.com:180/bol/topic?eu=118681&sctn=1> [Accessed 19 October 1999].
2.  World Health Organization. Trends in substance use and associated health problems. Fact sheet no. 127, August 1996. Geneva: World Health Organization, 1996.
3.  Breslow RA, Subar AF, Patterson BH, Block G. Trends in food intake: the 1987 and 1992 National Health Interview Surveys. Nutr Cancer 1997;28:86-92.
4.  Grant BF, Harford TC, Dawson DA, Chou P, Dufour M, Pickering R. Prevalence of DSM-IV alcohol abuse and dependence: United States, 1992. Alcohol Health Res World 1994;18: 243-48.
5.  Klatsky AL, Armstrong MA, Friedman GD. Alcohol and mortality. Ann Intern Med 1992; 117:646-54.
6.  Pearson TA. Alcohol and heart disease. AHA Science Advisory. Circulation 1996;94:3023-25.
7.  Gaziano JM, Buring JE, Breslow JL, et al. Moderate alcohol intake, increased levels of high-density lipoprotein and its subfractions, and decreased risk of myocardial infarction. N Engl J Med 1993;329:1829-34.
8.  Gordon T, Ernst N, Fisher M, Rifkind BM. Alcohol and high-density lipoprotein cholesterol. Circulation 1981;64(3 Pt 2):III63-III67.
9.  Criqui MH, Cowan LD, Tyroler HA, et al. Lipoproteins as mediators for the effects of alcohol consumption and cigarette smoking on cardiovascular mortality: Results from the Lipid Research Clinics Follow-up Study. Am J Epidemiol 1987;126:629-37.
10. Sane T, Nikkila EA, Taskinen MR, Valimaki M, Ylikahri R. Accelerated turnover of very low density lipoprotein triglycerides in chronic alcohol users. A possible mechanism for the up-regulation of high density lipoprotein by ethanol. Atherosclerosis 1984;53:185-93.
11. Jones DP, Losowsky MS, Davidson CS, Lieber CS. Effects of ethanol on plasma lipids in man. J Lab Clin Med 1963;62:675-82.
12. Taskinen M-R, Nikkilä EA. Nocturnal hypertriglyceridemia and hyperinsulinemia following moderate evening intake of alcohol. Acta Med Scand 1977;202:173-77.
13. Mishra L, Le N-A, Brown WV, Mezey E. Effect of acute intravenous alcohol on plasma lipoproteins in man. Metabolism 1991;40:1128-30.
14. Schneider J, Liesenfeld A, Mordasini R, et al. Lipoprotein fractions, lipoprotein lipase and hepatic triglyceride lipase during short-term and long-term uptake of ethanol in healthy subjects. Atherosclerosis 1985;57:281-91.
15. Pownall HJ. Dietary ethanol is associated with reduced lipolysis of intestinally derived lipoproteins. J Lipid Res 1994;35:2105-13.

16.     Pownall HJ, Ballantyne CM, Kimball KT, Simpson SL, Yeshurun D, Gotto AM Jr. Effect of moderate alcohol consumption on hypertriglyceridemia: a study in the fasting state. Arch Intern Med 1999;159:981-87.

17.     Talbot GD, Keating BM. Effects of preprandial whiskey on postalimentary lipemia. Geriatrics 1962;17:802-8.

18.     Barboriak JJ, Meade RC. Enhancement of alimentary lipemia by preprandial alcohol. Am J Med Sci 1968;255:245-51.

19.     Wilson DE, Schreibman PH, Brewster AC, Arky RA. The enhancement of alimentary lipemia by ethanol in man. J Lab Clin Med 1970;75:264-74.

20.     Superko HR. Effects of acute and chronic alcohol consumption on postprandial lipemia in healthy normotriglyceridemic men. Am J Cardiol 1992;69:701-4.

21.     Friedewald WT, Levy RI, Fredrickson DS. Estimation of the concentration of low-density lipoprotein cholesterol in plasma, without the use of the preparative ultracentrifuge. Clin Chem 1972;18:499-502.

22.     Bilheimer DW, Eisenberg S, Levy RI. The metabolism of very low density lipoprotein proteins. I. Preliminary in vitro and in vivo observations. Biochim Biophys Acta 1972;260: 212-21.

23.     Lindgren FT, Jensen LC, Hatch FT. The isolation and quantitative analysis of serum lipoproteins. In: Nelson GJ, editor. Blood lipids and lipoproteins: Quantitation, composition, and metabolism. New York: Wiley-Interscience, 1972:181-274.

24.     Egusa G, Brady DW, Grundy SM, Howard BV. Isopropanol precipitation method for the determination of apolipoprotein B specific activity and plasma concentrations during metabolic studies of very low density lipoprotein and low density lipoprotein apolipoprotein B. J Lipid Res 1983;24:1261-67.

25.     Goldberg CS, Tall AR, Krumholz S. Acute inhibition of hepatic lipase and increase in plasma lipoproteins after alcohol intake. J Lipid Res 1984;25:714-20.

26.     Taskinen MR, Valimaki M, Nikkila EA, Kuusi T, Ylikahri R. Sequence of alcohol-induced initial changes in plasma lipoproteins (VLDL and HDL) and lipolytic enzymes in humans. Metabolism 1985;34:112-19.

27.     Nishiwaki M, Ishikawa T, Ito T, et al. Effects of alcohol on lipoprotein lipase, hepatic lipase, cholesteryl ester transfer protein, and lecithin:cholesterol acyltransferase in high-density lipoprotein cholesterol elevation. Atherosclerosis 1994;111:99-109.

28.     Jones DP, Perman ES, Lieber CS. Free fatty acid turnover and triglyceride metabolism after ethanol ingestion in man. J Lab Clin Med 1965;66:804-13.

29.     Tobias H, Dawson AM. Free fatty acid mobilization and plasma triglyceride clearance in alcoholic hyperlipemia (abstract). Gastroenterology 1966;50:393.

30.     Nikkila EA, Taskinen MR, Huttunen JK. Effect of acute ethanol load on postheparin plasma lipoprotein lipase and hepatic lipase activities and intravenous fat tolerance. Horm Metab Res 1978;10:220-23.

31.     Verdy M, Gattereau A. Ethanol, lipase activity, and serum-lipid level. Am J Clin Nutr 1967; 20:997-1003.

ALCOHOL, COAGULATION, AND FIBRINOLYSIS

Cornelis Kluft

## Introduction

The interest in the effects of alcohol consumption on coagulation and fibrinolysis stems from the observations of a reduced risk of cardiovascular disease for moderate users of alcohol. The participation of thrombi in myocardial infarction and the fibrin hypothesis for vascular wall thickening indicate to evaluate the effects of alcohol on the fibrin forming and dissolving systems.

As recently reviewed by Hendriks and van der Gaag [1], several effects of alcohol on haemostatic variables and associations between alcohol use and haemostatic variables have been documented. An important question is whether or not such associations or changes are of mechanistic importance for the risk of cardiovascular disease. As discussed in this manuscript, answers to this question concerning fibrinogen and plasminogen activator inhibitor 1 (PAI-1) require further experimental and epidemiological studies in genetically homogeneous subgroups and with detailed definition of the clinical phenotype.

### Genetic Polymorphisms and Response to Environment

Our genome displays a large number of differences between individuals and is estimated to have an average frequency of one difference in 200 base pairs. We can distinguish several categories for these differences. Many are neutral but some cause defects which have a great impact on our health, but remain at a very low population frequency ($<<1\%$) due to selection. One important category contains the differences with a modest impact on health, that have a high frequency (1-50%) but may acquire importance in relation to the environment. Such differences frequently are variations in the promotor region of a gene causing a difference in the regulation of expression in response to environmental changes or differences. Such response polymorphisms are known for both fibrinogen and PAI-1. It appears relevant to consider such polymorphisms when discussing the effects of alcohol consumption.

A recent observation on PAI-1 can serve to illustrate the principle of response polymorphisms. The gene for PAI-1 contains a common polymorphism with either a stretch of four Gs or five Gs in the promotor region. The frequency of both is about equal. The 4G stretch is relatively insensitive to repression with the consequence that in cases when PAI-1

*R. Paoletti et al. (eds.), Moderate Alcohol Consumption and Cardiovascular Disease, 53–60.*
© 2000 *Kluwer Academic Publishers and Fondazione Giovanni Lorenzini. Printed in the Netherlands.*

synthesis is stimulated the carriers of the 4G allele show a stronger increase [2]. This implies that in carriers of 4G the inhibition of fibrinolysis shows in the case of a situation of stimulation a relative imbalance to the activity of fibrinolysis compared to the 5G carriers and potentially induces a tendency to prolong the persistence of the fibrin.

In patients with meningococcal disease this has been shown to be of relevance for the risk of septic shock. Firstly, it was shown that the 4G carriers had higher PAI-1 levels and secondly these carriers had a higher risk of septic shock [3,4]. This demonstrates the importance of response genetics for specific disease situations.

## Clinical End-Points and Intervention

Traditionally many diseases have been categorized by clinical criteria and by organ specificity. To acquire a good match with a genetic and mechanistic approach requires however the definition of (sub)groups of disease with homogeneous pathogenesis. An interesting example of such matching concerns the research on a mutation in the clotting factor V. The mutation discovered in Leiden is called factor V Leiden [5] and shows a prevalence in Caucasian populations of 3-5%. The relatively high frequency of this clotting defect has facilitated studies on the impact of this specific defect on clinical phenotypes. Firstly, it was observed that this anticlotting defect was associated mostly with venous thrombotic disease and less or not at all with various types of arterial thrombotic disease such as myocardial infarction. Such an observation was also made for defects in other coagulation and fibrinolysis factors [6]. Secondly, it was observed that association with deep venous thrombosis was stronger than with superficial thrombophlebitis and pulmonary embolism, emphasizing that these phenotypes should be considered separately [7]. These observations demand an increased attention to detailed clinical and diagnostic characterisation of patients and phenotypes. In epidemiology the past definitions of the clinical endpoints may in this respect be insufficient for the future.

Another example may illustrate the possibility of mechanistic heterogeneity that could determine the potential effects of treatment and preventive measures. In the Thrombosis prevention trial in the UK the effect of low-intensity oral anticoagulation, aspirin and the combination was investigated for their effect on myocardial infarction [8]. It was shown that the first two treatments were effective, but with respect to different clinical end-points: Aspirin for nonfatal myocardial infarction and oral anticoagulation for fatal myocardial infarction. Interestingly, the combination treatment was effective for about twice the number of patients as for the separate treatments. This strongly suggests at least two different pathogenetic mechanisms and effects of each treatment only predominantly for one of these two mechanisms.

## Fibrinogen

An increased fibrinogen blood level is one of the main established haemostatic risk variables for cardiovascular disease [9]. The gene variation at -455G/A (rare allele, 19%)

is associated with an increased response to trauma [10,11], possibly due to its complete linkage disequilibrium with the -148C/T polymorphism which is located adjacent to the interleukin-6 responsive element of the fibrinogen-beta gene promotor. Also the baseline concentration of fibrinogen is different for the various genotypes of -455G/A. The question arises whether the plasma concentration itself is the etiological factor or a marker of the genetic variation for responsiveness in acute situations, or both. The association between the -455G/A polymorphism and disease has been evaluated in several epidemiological studies and intervention studies. Surprisingly, no association between the genotype and myocardial infarction was observed [cf 12], or only in specific groups [13]. Instead an association between the genotype and the progression of luminal narrowing was observed [14,15]. In the latter situation the plasma level was not informative. It suggests that the transient responsiveness of fibrinogen to trauma / inflammation is relevant to the progressive deterioration in vascular wall pathology and not to clot formation during myocardial infarction.

As reviewed by Hendriks and van der Gaag [1] twelve recent studies have reported an association between alcohol consumption and fibrinogen levels. Eight of the twelve studies reviewed by them have shown an inverse or a partially inverse association. More recent and other studies confirm the inverse relationship [16-20] and further reports suggest the specificity of the relationship since in elderly subjects no relation at all has been found in three countries [21] and no association was found for beer and cider [20]. Limited experimental studies are available, but these indicate a reduction in fibrinogen due to the alcohol component [22,23].

In view of the above genetic considerations, the question arises of whether the association is additionally confined to specific fibrinogen genotypes. Genetic epidemiological studies are not known. For experimental studies on the effects of alcohol a genetic sampling frame may be used and different genotypes studied separately. The question that may be addressed is whether the increase in fibrinogen after a period of strenuous exercise as studied by Montgomery et al. [10] is genotype-specifically modified by alcohol.

A potential mechanism by which alcohol may reduce fibrinogen is its anti-inflammatory effect. The acute phase marker C-reactive protein (CRP) shows a distinct continuous level indicative of continuous low grade activity in the repair and inflammatory systems [24]. These levels are relatively stable in individuals and show a relatively strong correlation with fibrinogen levels. This is an indication that low grade inflammation is a major determinant of habitual fibrinogen levels.

It would be intriguing to know whether the association between CRP and fibrinogen is genotype-specific. A recent study on intima-media thickness in the Rotterdam Study showed a significant association between CRP and intima-media thickness (unpublished). This further supports a role of fibrinogen in vascular wall pathology.

A very recent report by Koenig et al. shows that moderate alcohol consumption is associated with reduced CRP levels [25]. In fact the analysis of the healthy population from the MONICA study shows a U-shaped pattern of CRP similar to the risk curves between alcohol and cardiovascular disease. These associations between alcohol use and CRP might be due to effects on the cytokines TNF-alpha and interleukin-6 capable of inducing CRP synthesis. Indeed, the effect of alcohol on the cytokine networks has been reported, as summarized by Deaciuc [26]. It has for example been shown in animals that ethanol reduces peak serum TNF-alpha levels [27] and the *ex vivo* proinflammatory cytokine expression of alveolar macrophages [28] upon a challenge.

Earlier Mendall et al. [29] reported associations between alcohol use and blood cytokine levels with a decreased level of TNF-alpha and increased level of interleukin-6 in humans. These observations on blood levels may well be explained by the increased clearance of TNF-alpha and decreased clearance of interleukin-6 as observed in alcohol-fed animals [30].

These studies indicate that alcohol produces an effect on inflammatory reactions which deserves further exploration and confirmation.

It can be concluded that the epidemiological observations on an inverse relationship between moderate alcohol use and fibrinogen blood levels require further mechanistic elucidation with the option that the alcohol effects are mediated through an anti-inflammatory effect and are genotype-specific. When the effect is genotype-specific a causal role of fibrinogen is strongly supported. With regard to the clinical effect, the effects of alcohol should be further evaluated specifically on vascular wall pathology, for instance on intima-media thickening.

## PAI-1/t-PA

PAI-1 is one of the main inhibitors of fibrinolysis and increased levels are associated with an increased risk of myocardial infarction [9]. The genetic variation in the promotor region (see above) is associated with baseline blood levels and with the response to acute trauma [2,3] and chronic situations such as higher lipid and glucose [31,32]. The genetic variant 4G is associated with higher risk of myocardial infarction as recently evaluated in a meta-analysis [33]. We observed that the risk is particularly strong in smokers [34]: smoking increases PAI-1.

For PAI-1 we have observed a perplexing strong increase acutely after alcohol consumption [35]. Levels went up 5-10 fold after 4 glasses of beverage containing alcohol, beer, wine, or Dutch gin. The effect was transient and PAI-1 reverted to normal the morning after the evening experiment. The increase in PAI-1 was accompanied by a decrease in active tissue-type plasminogen activator, and a decrease in plasmin-antiplasmin complexes. Clearly a fibrinolytic shut-down in the circulation was obtained. The eight individuals in the study performed in random order all "treatments" and it could be observed that the increase was reasonably reproducible between alcohol events (Spearman's coefficient between 0.57 and 0.81 for all combinations of response expressed as area under the curve). The responses between individuals showed a broad range when the area under the curve was considered, varying a factor 2-3. It is possible though not yet investigated that this is related to the 4G/5G polymorphism. Also, the effect of beer was in seven out of the eight individuals stronger than that of wine or gin.

It is difficult to reconcile this seemingly negative effect of alcohol on fibrinolysis with a reduced risk of cardiovascular disease. In view of the expectation that the response will be different for 5G carriers a check should be made in epidemiology that 5G carriers have a larger reduction in cardiovascular risk with moderate alcohol consumption.

In addition to the increase in PAI-1 activity and antigen, t-PA antigen is also increased during the post-alcohol period [35]. Apparently, PAI-1 increase dominates in view of the reduction in t-PA activity. However, an induced increase in t-PA cannot be concluded with confidence from the increased circulating levels of t-PA antigen. Reduced clearance of the t-PA and/or t-PA/PAI-1 complex may also explain the observed increase in t-PA antigen. On the other hand studies on t-PA synthesis by endothelial cells provide evidence of a possible increased synthesis of t-PA [36-40].

Although the balance between t-PA and PAI-1 seems to be unfavorable for the circulating amount of active t-PA, it is not impossible that an increased production of t-PA, when occurring *in vivo*, is beneficial to the local effects and to the acute release of t-PA. It has been demonstrated *in vitro* that the acute release is proportional to the production rate of t-PA [41], suggesting the possibility of a beneficial effect of alcohol in acute situations. This option can be experimentally verified by acute release experiments such as with the techniques of Jern et al. [42].

For the PAI-1/t-PA effects it is difficult to judge whether the net effect of alcohol is positive or negative and whether there is a time effect. Our original investigations on the acute effects of alcohol on PAI-1 and t-PA suggested the possibility that the differences in time scale of these effects created an increase in fibrinolytic activity in the circulation on the morning following alcohol use with the evening meal [1,35]. This coincides with the circadian increase of risk in the morning and might be the right moment for such a potentially protective increase in fibrinolysis. This remains however only a speculation.

# References

1.     Hendriks HFJ , Gaag, van der MS. Alcohol, coagulation and fibrinolysis. In: 1998 Alcohol and cardiovascular diseases. Wiley: Chichester (Novartis Foundation Symposium 216), 1998: 111-24.

2.     Eriksson P, Nilsson L, Karpe F, Hamsten A. Very-low-density lipoprotein response element in the promotor region of the human plasminogen activator inhibitor-1 gene: Implicated in the impaired fibrinolysis of hypertriglyceridemia. Arterioscler Thromb Vasc Biol 1998;18:20-26.

3.     Westendorp RG, Hottenga JJ, Slagboom PE. Variation in plasminogen-activator-inhibitor-1 gene and risk of meningococcal septic shock. Lancet 1999;354:561-63.

4.     Hermans PW, Hibberd ML, Booy R, et al. 4G/5G promotor polymorphism in the plasminogen-activator-inhibitor-1 gene and outcome of meningococcal disease. Meningococcal Research Group. Lancet 1999;354:556-60.

5.     Bertina RM, Koeleman BPC, Koster T, et al. Mutation in blood coagulation factor V associated with resistance to activated protein C. Nature 1994;369:64-67.

6.     Kluft C, Iacoviello L, Genetics of myocardial infarction: Haemocoagulative aspects. Cardiologia 1997;42(Suppl.3):697-700.
7.     Manten B, Westendorp RGJ, Koster T, Reitsma P. Risk factor profiles in patients with different clinical manifestations of venous thromboembolism: A focus on the factor V Leiden mutation. Thromb Haemos 1996;76:510-13.
8.     The Medical Research Council's General Practice Research Framework. Thrombosis Prevention trial: Randomised trial of low-intensity oral anticoagulation with warfarin and low-dose aspirin in the primary prevention of ischaemic heart disease in men at increased risk. Lancet 1998;351:233-41.
9.     Iacoviello L, Zito F, Di Castelnuovo A, de Maat M, Kluft C, Donati MB. Contribution of factor VII, fibrinogen and fibrinolytic components to the risk of ischaemic cardiovascular disease: Their genetic determinants. Fibrinolysis & Proteolysis 1998; 12:259-76.
10.    Montgomery HE, Clarkson P, Nwose OM, et al. The acute rise in plasma fibrinogen concentration with exercise is influenced by the G-453-A polymorphism of the beta-fibrinogen gene. Arterioscler Thromb Vasc Biol 1996;16:386-91.
11.    Ferrer-Antunes C, de Maat MP, Palmeiro A, Pimentel J, Fernandes V. Association between polymorphisms in the fibrinogen alpha- and beta-genes on the post-trauma fibrinogen increase. Thromb Res 1998;92:207-12.
12.    Van der Bom JG, de Maat MPM, Bots ML, et al. Elevated plasma fibrinogen. Cause or consequence of cardiovascular disease? Arterioscler Thromb Vasc Biol 1998;18: 621-25.
13.    Zito F, Di Castelnuovo A, Amore C, D'Orazio A, Donati MB, Iacoviello L. Bcl I polymorphism in the fibrinogen beta-chain gene is associated with the risk of familial myocardial infarction by increasing plasma fibrinogen levels. A case-control study in a sample of GISSI-2 patients. Arterioscler Thromb Vasc Biol 1997;17:3489-94.
14.    De Maat MPM, Kastelein JJP, Jukema JW, et al. -455G/A polymorphism of the beta-fibrinogen gene is associated with the progression of coronary atherosclerosis in symptomatic men. Proposed role for an acute-phase reaction pattern of fibrinogen. Arterioscler Thromb Vasc Biol 1998;18:265-71.
15.    Schmidt H, Schmidt R, Niederkorn K, et al. Beta-fibrinogen gene polymorphism (C148-T) is associated with carotid atherosclerosis: Results of the Austrian Stroke Prevention Study. Arterioscler Thromb Vasc Biol 1998;18:487-92.
16.    Woodward M, Lowe GD, Rumley A, et al. Epidemiology of coagulation factors, inhibitors and activation markers: The Third Glasgow MONICA Survey. II. Relationships to cardiovascular risk factors and prevalent cardiovascular disease. Br J Haematol 1997;97:785-97.
17.    Margaglione M, Cappucci G, Colaizzo D, et al. Fibrinogen plasma levels in an apparently healthy general population—relation to environmental and genetic determinants. Thromb Haemost 1998;80:805-10.
18.    Scarabin PY, Aillaud MF, Amouyel P, et al. Associations of fibrinogen, factor VII and PAI-1 with baseline findings among 10,500 male participants in a prospective study of myocardial infarction-the PRIME Study. Prospective Epidemiological Study of Myocardial infarction. Thromb Haemost 1998;80:749-56.
19.    Pitsavos C, Skoumas J, Dernellis J, et al. Influence of biological factors on lipid and fibrinogen measurements in young men. An epidemiological study in 2009 recruits. Eur Heart J 1998;19:1642-47.
20.    Mennen LI, Balkau B, Vol S, Caces E, Eschwege E. Fibrinogen: A possible link between

alcohol consumption and cardiovascular disease? DESIR Study Group. Arterioscler Thromb Vasc Biol 1999;19:887-92.

21. Bijnen FC, Feskens EJ, Giampaoli S, et al. Haemostatic parameters and lifestyle factors in elderly men in Italy and The Netherlands. Thromb Haemost 1996;76:411-16.

22. Dimmitt SB, Rakic V, Puddey IB, et al. The effects of alcohol on coagulation and fibrinolytic factors: A controlled trial. Blood Coagul Fibrinolysis 1998;9:39-45.

23. Pellegrini N, Pareti FI, Stabile F, Brusamolino A, Simonetti P. Effects of moderate consumption of red wine on platelet aggregation and haemostatic variables in healthy volunteers. Eur J Clin Nutr 1996;50:209-13.

24. De Maat MPM, Haverkate F, Kluft C. C-reactive protein: A cardiovascular risk factor. Report on the CRP hot-topic workshop October 1, 1997. Fibrinolysis & Proteolysis 1998;12:323-27.

25. Koenig W, Sund M, Froehlich M, et al. C-reactive protein, a sensitive marker of inflammation, predicts future risk of coronary heart disease in initially healthy middle-aged men. Circulation 1999;99:237-42.

26. Deaciuc IV. Alcohol and cytokine networks. Alcohol 1997;14:421-30.

27. Nelson S, Bagdy GJ, Bainton BG, Summer WR. The effects of acute and chronic alcoholism on tumour necrosis factor and the inflammatory response. J Infect Dis 1989;1609:422-29.

28. Standiford TJ, Danforth JM. Ethanol feeding inhibits proinflammatory cytokine expression from murine alveolar macrophages ex vivo. Alcohol Clin Exp Res 1997;21:1212-17.

29. Mendall MA, Patel P, Asante M, et al. Relation of serum cytokine concentrations to cardiovascular risk factors and coronary heart disease. Heart 1997;78:273-77.

30. Deaciuc IV, Alappat JM, McDonough KH, D'Souza NB. Effect of chronic alcohol consumption by rats on tumor necrosis factor-alpha and interleukin-6clearance in vivo and by the isolated, perfused liver. Biochem Pharmacol 1996;52:891-99.

31. Panahloo A, Mohamed-Ali V, Lane A, Green F, Humphries SE, Yudkin JS. Determinants of plasminogen activator inhibitor 1 activity in treated NIDDM and its relation to a polymorphism in the plasminogen activator inhibitor 1 gene. Diabetes 1995;44:37-42.

32. Mansfield MW, Stickland MH, Grant PJ. Environmental and genetic factors in relation to elevated circulating levels of plasminogen activator inhibitor-1 in Caucasian patients with non-insulin-dependent diabetes mellitus. Thromb Haemost 1995;74: 842-47.

33. Iacoviello L, Burzotta F, Di Castelnuovo A, Zito F, Marchioli R, Donati MB. The 4G/5G polymorphism of PAI-1 promoter gene and the risk of myocardial infarction: A meta-analysis. Thromb Haemost 1998;80:1029-30.

34. Van der Bom JG, Bots ML, Haverkate F, et al. Smoking modifies the risk of myocardial infarction associated with the 4G5G polymorphism at the PAI-1 gene locus. Thesis, Erasmus University, Rotterdam, 1997.

35. Hendriks HFJ, Veenstra J, Velthuis-teWierik EJM, Schaafsma G, Kluft C. Effect of moderate dose of alcohol with evening meal on fibrinolytic factors. Br Med J 1994; 306:1003-6.

36. Grenett HE, Aikens ML, Torres JA, et al. Ethanol transcriptionally upregulates t-PA and u-PA gene expression in cultured human endothelial cells. Alcohol Clin Exp Res 1998;22:849-53.

37. Miyamoto A, Yang S-X, Laufs U, Ruan X-L, Liao JK. Activation of guanine nucleotide-

binding proteins and induction of endothelial tissue-type plasminogen activator gene transcription by alcohol. J Biol Chem 1999;274:12055-60.

38.    Aikens ML, Grenett HE, Benza RL, Tabengwa EM, Davis GC, Booyse FM. Alcohol-induced upregulation of plasminogen activators and fibrinolytic activity in cultured human endothelial cells. Alcohol Clin Exp Res 1998;22:375-81.

39.    Aikens ML, Benza RL, Grenett HE, et al. Ethanol increases surface-localized fibrinolytic activity in cultured endothelial cells. Alcohol Clin Exp Res 1997;21:1471-78.

40.    Venkov CD, Su M, Shyr Y, Vaughan DE. Ethanol-induced alterations in the expression of endothelial-derived fibrinolytic components. Fibrinolysis & Proteolysis 1997;11:115-18.

41.    Van den Eijnden-Schrauwen Y, Kooistra T, de Vries RE, Emeis JJ. Studies on the acute release of tissue-type plasminogen activator from human endothelial cells in vitro and in rats in vivo: Evidence for a dynamic storage pool. Blood 1995;85: 3510-17.

42.    Jern C, Ladenvall P, Wall U, Jern S. Gene polymorphism of t-PA is associated with forearm vascular release rate of t-PA. Arterioscler Thromb Vasc Biol 1999;19:454-59.

# Moderate Alcohol Consumption, Insulin Resistance, and Cardiovascular Disease

Gerald M. Reaven

## Introduction

Epidemiological studies [1-6] have repeatedly demonstrated that mild-to-moderate alcohol consumption is associated with a decrease in cardiovascular disease (CVD). Despite these observations, the relationship between alcohol and CVD has received relatively little attention, presumably because of the obvious disastrous consequences of excessive alcohol consumption. However, the untoward effects of too much alcohol should not prevent consideration of the beneficial effects described in individuals consuming amounts of alcohol below the levels of intake leading to liver disease, pancreatitis, etc.

The goal of this presentation will be to review the metabolic changes identified in light-to-moderate drinkers that might account for their decreased risk of CVD. In particular, attention will be focused on the possibility that insulin sensitivity is enhanced in individuals consuming light-to-moderate amounts of alcohol, and this effect contributes to the decrease in CVD risk.

## Alcohol Consumption, Dyslipidemia, And CVD

A low high density lipoprotein (HDL) cholesterol concentration is a well-recognized CVD risk factor [7,8], and there is evidence that the beneficial effect of moderate alcohol consumption on CVD is mediated via is its ability to raise HDL cholesterol concentrations [5,6,9-16]. Although differences of opinion exist as to whether alcohol consumption is associated with increases in $HDL_2$ [14], or $HDL_3$ [11,13], or both [15,16], there is general agreement that there is a direct relationship between HDL cholesterol concentration and alcohol intake. In general, high HDL cholesterol concentrations tend to be accompanied by lower plasma triglyceride (TG) concentrations. However, this doesn't seem to be the case as regards the changes in HDL cholesterol concentration associated with alcohol consumption. Indeed, it is generally assumed that the greater the intake of alcohol, the higher the plasma TG concentration. However, the generalization may not apply to individuals consuming < 30 g of alcohol per day, in which case plasma TG concentrations may be similar, or lower, than in abstainers [15-17].

*R. Paoletti et al. (eds.), Moderate Alcohol Consumption and Cardiovascular Disease, 61–66.*
© 2000 *Kluwer Academic Publishers and Fondazione Giovanni Lorenzini. Printed in the Netherlands.*

## Alcohol and HDL Cholesterol Metabolism

Given evidence of a direct relationship between alcohol intake and HDL cholesterol concentration, it is surprising how little information is available concerning the effect of alcohol intake on HDL metabolism. For example, there is evidence from kinetic studies that the fractional catabolic rate (FCR) of apoA-I/HDL is accentuated in individuals with endogenous hypertriglyceridemia [18-20], type 2 diabetes [21], and essential hypertension [22]. Furthermore, it appears that the more rapid the FCR of apoA-1/HDL, the lower the HDL cholesterol concentration [21-23]. Thus, it could be speculated that the increase in HDL cholesterol concentrations associated with mild to moderate alcohol consumption is due to a decrease in the FCR of apoA-1/HDL. Unfortunately, there does not appear to be published data to support, or rule out, this possibility.

If it is assumed that higher HDL cholesterol concentrations in users of alcohol are due to decreases in the FCR of apoA-1/HDL, it is necessary to ask why this is the case. In this context it should be noted that syndromes associated with increases in the FCR of apoA-1/HDL, i.e. hypertension, hypertriglyceridemia, and type 2 diabetes [18-22], are associated with insulin resistance and compensatory hyperinsulinemia [24]. and is evidence of a direct relationship between plasma insulin concentrations and the FCR of apoA-1/HDL [21-23]. Thus, it is possible that insulin sensitivity is enhanced in association with alcohol intake, and this change leads to a decrease in the FCR of apoA-1/HDL, and higher HDL cholesterol concentrations.

## Alcohol and Insulin Sensitivity

To evaluate the possibility that mild-to-moderate alcohol intake is associated with enhanced insulin sensitivity, plasma lipid and lipoprotein concentrations, plasma glucose and insulin responses to an oral glucose challenge, and insulin-mediated glucose disposal rates were compared in 40 healthy volunteers—20 individuals who were light-to-moderate consumers of alcohol and 20 nondrinkers. Habitual intake of alcohol was estimated by questionnaire, based on an average estimated alcohol content of 10, 4, 40, and 20% (weight), respectively, for wine, beer, spirits, and mixed. Light-to-moderate drinking was defined as consumption of 10-30 g of alcohol per day, an amount roughly equivalent to 1-3 drinks/day.

The 20 nondrinkers were healthy volunteers who stated that they never consumed alcohol (n = 14), or only used it on rare occasions (n = 6). They were otherwise identical to the 20 drinkers in terms of gender distribution, age, body mass index, ratio of waist to hip girth, family history of hypertension or type 2 diabetes, and estimates of habitual physical activity. Finally, only 2 of the 40 participants smoked.

The total integrated glucose response to a 75 g oral glucose challenge was significantly lower in light-to-moderate drinkers ($17.8 \pm 0.8$ versus $19.8 \pm 0.9$ mM/h, $p < 0.02$). The difference in the total integrated plasma insulin response between the two groups was greater, and was significantly lower ($p < 0.01$) in light-to-moderate drinkers ($600 \pm 65$ pM/h) than in nondrinkers ($1,075 \pm 160$ pM/h).

Insulin-mediated glucose uptake was estimated by a modification [25] of the insulin suppression test originally described by our research group [26]. This approach is based on the continuous intravenous infusion for 180 minutes of somatostatin (5 µg/min), insulin (25 mU/m²/min), and glucose (240 mg/m²/min). Venous blood samples are every 10 minutes during the last 30 minutes for measurement of plasma glucose and insulin concentrations, and the mean value for these four measurements used to calculate the steady-state plasma insulin (SSPI) and steady-state plasma glucose (SSPG) concentrations.

Despite the similarity of the SSPI concentrations in the two groups (~300 pmol/L), the SSPG concentrations were significantly higher in light-to-moderate drinkers ($10.7 \pm 1.2$ versus $6.7 \pm 0.8$ mmol/L, $p < 0.01$). Thus, individuals who abstain from the alcohol were less able to dispose of the infused glucose load, i.e. they were relatively insulin resistant as compared to light to moderate consumers of alcohol.

In addition to being more insulin sensitive, light-to-moderate drinkers had significantly higher ($p < 0.02$) HDL cholesterol concentrations ($1.46 \pm 0.08$ versus $1.25 \pm 0.08$ mmol/L) than nondrinkers. However, there was no increase in either LDL cholesterol ($2.56 \pm 0.18$ versus $2.49 \pm 0.15$ mmol/L) or triglyceride ($1.18 \pm 0.12$ versus $1.21 \pm 0.11$ mmol/L) concentrations in those consuming alcoholic beverages.

These results show that light-to-moderate drinkers are relatively more insulin sensitive, and have lower plasma insulin levels, than do nondrinkers. Because the two experimental groups were well-matched in age, sex distribution, and degree of obesity and habitual physical activity, i.e. variables known to affect insulin action and insulin concentration, it seems reasonable to conclude that the difference in alcohol intake was responsible for the observed changes in insulin metabolism. These results are also quite consistent with published information that plasma insulin concentrations are lower in population-based studies of both men and women [15-17,27]. Thus, there is substantial evidence that light-to-moderate consumers of alcohol are more insulin sensitive than are individuals who do not use alcoholic beverages.

The conclusion that light-to-moderate drinkers are more insulin sensitive than abstainers is not in conflict with previous publications showing that the acute administration of large amounts of alcohol decreased insulin-mediated glucose disposal [28-30]. These studies were performed in a relatively small number of individuals (7, 10, and 6 in references 28-30, respectively), and large amounts of alcohol were administered intravenously over quite short time periods, i.e. total doses ranging from 22 g in 7 hours to ~ 60 g in 30 minutes. Obviously, the amounts are greatly in excess of the daily 10-30 g of alcohol consumed by the light-to-moderate drinkers in this study.

The evidence that enhanced insulin sensitivity was present in light-to-moderate drinkers does not mean that alcohol consumption should be encouraged to improve insulin-mediated glucose disposal; the dangers of excessive alcohol intake are well appreciated and need not be repeated. Furthermore, the changes in insulin-mediated glucose disposal and plasma insulin concentration noted in light-to-moderate drinkers are not necessarily caused by alcohol consumption, *per se*. Although we tried to take into account all relevant variables known to affect insulin action and glucose tolerance, some other variable, present in drinkers and not nondrinkers, was possibly responsible for the changes noted. However, even if this were the case, it would not alter the fact that nondrinkers were relatively insulin resistant, glucose intolerant, and hyperinsulinemic compared to light-to-moderate drinkers.

## Conclusion

There is substantial evidence that light-to-moderate alcohol consumption is associated with: 1) decreased risk of CVD; 2) higher HDL cholesterol concentrations; 3) enhanced insulin sensitivity and lower plasma insulin concentrations. It is possible with this information to construct a coherent formulation that links the four variables together in the following manner. As a group, light-to-moderate drinkers are more insulin sensitive and have lower insulin concentrations than nondrinkers. The more insulin sensitive an individual, the lower their insulin concentration, the higher their HDL cholesterol [31,32]. In the case of light-to-moderate drinkers, this is presumably related to a decrease in the FCR of apoA-1/HDL. However whatever the mechanism responsible for the relationship between insulin and HDL cholesterol metabolism, the higher HDL cholesterol concentrations in light-to-moderate drinkers should decrease their risk of CVD.

Finally, although the hypothesis outlined above links mild-to-moderate alcohol consumption to decreased risk of CVD by modulation of HDL cholesterol concentration, it should be remembered that the lower glucose and insulin concentrations seen in light-to-moderate drinkers have also been identified as decreasing risk of CVD in nondiabetic individuals [33-37]. Thus, there are multiple reasons why CVD risk is lower in individuals consuming mild to moderate amounts of alcohol. It seems reasonable to suggest that we need to learn much more about this relationship, and how this information could be used to reduce CVD risk.

## References

1.      Marmot MG, Rose G, Shipley MJ, Thomas BJ. Alcohol and mortality: A U-shaped curve. Lancet 1981;I:580-83.
2.      Gordon T, Kannel WB. Drinking habits and cardiovascular disease. The Framingham study. Am Heart J 1983;105:667-73.
3.      Stampfer MJ, Colditz GA, Willet WC, Speizer FE, Hennekens CH. A prospective study of moderate alcohol consumption and the risk of coronary disease and stroke in women. N Engl J Med 1988;319:267-73.
4.      Jackson R, Scragg R, Beaglehole R. Alcohol consumption and risk of coronary heart disease. Br Med J 1991;303:211-15.
5.      Steinberg D, Pearson TA, Kuller LH. Alcohol and atherosclerosis. Ann Intern Med 1991; 114: 967-76.
6.      Suh I, Shaten BJ, Cutler JA, Kuller LH. Alcohol use and mortality from coronary heart disease: The role of high-density lipoprotein cholesterol. Ann Intern Med 1992;116:881-87.
7.      Miller GJ, Miller NE. Plasma HDL concentration and development of ischaemic heart

disease. Lancet 1975;I:16-19

8.    Gordon T, Castelli WP, Hjortland MC. High density lipoprotein as a protective factor against coronary heart disease: The Framingham Study. Am J Med 1977;62:707-14.

9.    Belfrage P, Berge B, Hagerstrand J, Nilsson-Ehle P, Tornqvist H, Wiebe T. Alteration of lipid metabolism in healthy volunteers during long term ethanol intake. Eur J Clin Invest 1977;7:127-31.

10.   Thornton J, Symes C, Heaton K. Moderate alcohol intake reduces bile cholesterol saturation and raises HDL cholesterol. Lancet 1983;u:819-22.

11.   Haskell WI, Camargo C, Williams PT, Vranizan KH, Kraus RM, Lindgren FT. The effect of cessation and resumption of moderate alcohol intake on serum high density lipoprotein subfractions: A controlled study. N Engl J Med 1984;310:805-10.

12.   Burr ML, Fehily AM, Butland BK, Bolton CH, Eastham RD. Alcohol and high density lipoprotein cholesterol: A randomized controlled trial. Br J Nutr 1986;56:81-86.

13.   Diehl AK, Fuller JM, Mattock MB, Salter AH, el-Gohar R, Keen H. The relationship of high density lipoproteins to alcohol consumption, and other lifestyle factors, and coronary heart disease. Atherosclerosis 1988;69:145-53.

14.   Miller NE, Bolton CH, Hayes TM, Bainton D, Yarnell JWG, Baker IA. Associations of alcohol consumption with plasma high density lipoprotein cholesterol and its major subfractions: The Caerphilly and Speedwell collaborative heart disease studies. J Epidemiol Community Health 1988;42:220-25.

15.   Razay G, Heaton KW, Bolton CH, Hughes AO. Alcohol consumption and its relation to cardiovascular risk factors in British women. Br Med J 1992;301:80-83.

16.   Razay G, Heaton KW. Alcohol consumption and cardiovascular risk factors in middle aged men. Cardiovascular Risk Factors 1995;5:200-5

17.   Facchini, F, Chen Y-DI, Reaven GM. Light to moderate alcohol intake is associated with enhanced insulin sensitivity. Diabetes Care 1994;17:115-19.

18.   Fidge N, Nestel P, Toshitsugu I, Reardon M, Billington T. Turnover of apoproteins A-I and A-II of high density lipoprotein and the relationship to other lipoproteins in normal and hyperlipidemic individuals. Metabolism 1980;29:643-53.

19.   Magill P, Rao SN, Miller NE, et al. Relationships between the metabolism of high-density and very-low-density lipoproteins in man: Studies of apolipoprotein kinetics and adipose tissue lipoprotein lipase activity. Eur J Clin Invest 1982;12:113-20.

20.   Schaefer EJ, Zech LA, Jenkins LL, et al. Human apolipoprotein A-I and A-II metabolism J Lipid Res 1982;23:850-62.

21.   Golay A, Zech L, Shi M-Z, Chiou Y-AM, Reaven GM, Chen Y-DI. High density lipoprotein (HDL) metabolism in noninsulin-dependent diabetes mellitus: Measurement of HDL turnover using tritiated HDL. J Clin Endocrinol Metab 1987;65:512-518.

22.   Chen Y-DI, Sheu WH-H, Swislocki ALM, Reaven GM. High density lipoprotein turnover in patients with hypertension. Hypertension 1991;17:386-93.

23.   Brinton EA, Eisenberg S, Breslow JL. Human HDL cholesterol levels are determined by apoA-I fractional catabolic rate, which correlates inversely with estimates of HDL particle size. Effects of gender, hepatic and lipoprotein lipases, triglyceride and insulin levels, and body fat distribution. Arterioscl Thromb 1994;14:707-20.

24.   Reaven GM. Role of insulin resistance in human disease. Diabetes 1988;37:1595-1607.

25.   Shen DC, Shieh SM, Fuh MT, Wu DA, Chen Y-DI, Reaven GM. Resistance to insulin-stimulated glucose uptake in patients with hypertension. J Clin Endocrinol Metab 1988;66:

580-83.

26.    Greenfield MS, Doberne L, Kraemer FB, Tobey TA, Reaven GM. Assessment of insulin
        resistance with the insulin-suppression test and the euglycemic clamp. Diabetes 1981;30:
        387-92.
27.    Kiechl S, Willeit J, Poewe W, Egger G, Overhollenzer F, Muggeo M. Insulin sensitivity
        and regular alcohol consumption; large, prospective, cross sectional population study
        (Bruneck study). Br Med J 1996;313:1040-44.
28.    Yki-Jarvinen H, Nikkila EA. Ethanol decreases glucose utilization in healthy men. J Clin
        Endocrinol Metab 1985;61:941-45.
29.    Yki-Jarvinen H, Koivisto VA, Ylikahri R, Taskinen M-R. Acute effects of ethanol and
        acetate on glucose kinetics in normal subjects. Am J Physiol 1988;254:E175-80.
30.    Shelmet JJ, Reichard GA, Skutches CL, Hoeldtke RD, Owen OE, Boden G. Ethanol
        causes acute inhibition of carbohydrate, fat, and protein oxidation and insulin resistance.
        J Clin Invest 1988;81;1137-45.
31.    Zavaroni I, Dall'Aglio E, Alpi O, et al. Evidence for an independent relationship between
        plasma insulin and concentration high-density lipoprotein cholesterol and triglyceride.
        Atherosclerosis 1985;55:256-66.
32.    Laws A, Reaven GM. Evidence for an independent relationship between insulin resistance
        and fasting plasma HDL-cholesterol, triglyceride and insulin concentrations. J Int Med.
        1992;231:25-30.
33.    Fuller JH, Shipley MJ, Rose G, Jarrett RJ, Keen H. Coronary heart disease and impaired
        glucose tolerance: The Whitehall Study. Lancet 1980;1:1373-76.
34.    Pyorala K, Savolainen E, Lehtovirta E, Punsar S, Siltanen P. Glucose tolerance and
        coronary heart disease: Helsinki Policemen Study. J Chronic Dis 1979;32:729-45.
35.    Ducimetiere P, Eschwege E, Papoz L, Richard JL, Claude JR, Rosselin G. Relationship
        of plasma insulin levels to the incidence of myocardial infarction and coronary heart
        disease mortality in a middle-aged population. Diabetologia 1980;19:205-10.
36.    Vaccaro O, Ruth KJ, Stamler J. Relationship of postload plasma glucose to mortality with
        19-yr follow-up. Diabetes Care 1992;13:1328-34.
37.    Depres J-P, Lamarche BM, Mauriege P, et al. Hyperinsulinemia as an independent risk
        factor for ischemic heart disease. N Engl J Med 1996;334:952-57.

# OXIDATIVE STRESS ASSOCIATED TO ALCOHOL CONSUMPTION

Emma A. Meagher

This chapter will discuss the potential role of alcohol as a mediator of oxidant injury and will suggest a mechanism whereby alcohol may be both beneficial and deleterious if consumed in modest amounts.

Alcohol-induced liver disease (ALD) is a common clinical entity and it represents approximately 45% of all cases of advanced liver disease. The exact mechanism whereby alcohol is deleterious to the liver is not clearly understood. The potential role that oxidant injury plays in the pathogenesis of alcoholic liver disease has received considerable scrutiny [1]. Alcohol ingestion, through the induction of the cytochrome P450 isozyme CPY2E1, may result in increased generation of reactive oxygen species (ROS) [2]. However, the ability to study this particular entity has been limited until recently by the inability to accurately measure oxidant activity *in vivo*. We have utilized measurement of urinary F2 isoprostanes as a measure of *in vivo* oxidant injury and *in vivo* free radical generation to study this particular question. Isoprostanes are free radical catalyzed products of arachidonic acid [3]. These are isomers of the more traditionally enzymatically formed eicosanoids. These compounds, in contrast with conventional indices of oxidant stress, are chemically stable, and may be measured by gas chromatography/mass spectrometry (GC/MS). Quantitation of isoprostanes in biological fluids reflects oxidant stress *in vivo*. One of these isoprostanes, $iPF_{2\alpha}$-III, is known to not only reflect free radical injury but also to have biological activity that includes vasoconstrictor effects, mitogenic activity, and to function as a platelet agonist. We have developed a methodology within our laboratory to measure isoprostanes including $iPF_{2\alpha}$-III by GC/MS. $iPF_{2\alpha}$-III is elevated in a variety of syndromes associated with oxidative stress including cigarette smoking, poisoning with paraquat, and during reperfusion following coronary ischemia [4-8]. Furthermore, we have demonstrated that in some of these systems oxidant injury can be modulated by antioxidant vitamin administration [6].

To address the hypothesis that alcohol concentrations compatible with social drinking result in increased oxidant stress we randomized healthy volunteers to receive different doses of alcohol. The dosing groups included placebo, 0.2, 0.3, 0.4, 0.6, and 0.9 grams of a 98% alcohol solution per kg body weight. Each study day was separated by a two-week interval. Alcohol was administered over a fifteen-minute period in a fasting state. Blood alcohol levels were measured at twenty-minute intervals during the first hour and then at 2, 3, 4, 6, 12, and 24 hours. In addition, urine was collected for isoprostane analysis.

67

*R. Paoletti et al. (eds.), Moderate Alcohol Consumption and Cardiovascular Disease, 67–72.*
© 2000 *Kluwer Academic Publishers and Fondazione Giovanni Lorenzini. Printed in the Netherlands.*

No alteration in isoprostane excretion was noted after administration of the control solution. In contrast, alcohol significantly increased peak urinary $iPF_{2\alpha}$-III excretion in a dose-dependent fashion. For example, the delta increase from baseline was $102 \pm 28$; $197 \pm 112$; $335 \pm 130$; and $401 \pm 120$ pg/mg creatinine after dosing with 0.3, 0.4, 0.6, and 0.9 g/kg ethanol, respectively. The corresponding peak plasma alcohol levels were $64.6 \pm 6.1$; $81.2 \pm 4.2$; $105 \pm 4.2$; and $130 \pm 5.6$ mg/dl.

To address the hypothesis that increased oxidant injury is a component of alcohol-induced liver disease, we measured isoprostane excretion in patients with alcohol-induced cirrhosis, in patients with a HCV cirrhosis, and in patients with liver disease of combined etiology. Hepatitis C is a common co-existent disease in patients with alcohol-induced liver disease. We compared these patients to age- and gender-matched healthy controls. All patients studied had similar degrees of liver impairment as assessed by the Childs Pugh Classification.

All patients with cirrhosis had elevated levels of urinary $iPF_{2\alpha}$-III when compared with controls ($663.5 \pm 95.2$ versus $127.2 \pm 7.9$ pg/mg creatinine; $p < 0.001$). Urinary $iPF_{2\alpha}$-III excretion was significantly increased in patients with HCV cirrhosis ($411.7 \pm 59.8$ pg/mg creatinine; $p < 0.001$). However, this increase was even more marked in those patients with ALD ($656.9 \pm 105.8$ pg/mg creatinine; $p < 0.001$) and those with combined disease ($921.9 \pm 120$; pg/mg creatinine; $p < 0.001$). There was no significant inter-individual variability among the three consecutive measurements for each individual studied.

Urinary excretion of the 2,3-dinor-5,6-dihydro-$iPF_{2\alpha}$-III metabolite was higher than that of the parent $iPF_{2\alpha}$-III in controls ($627 \pm 98.3$ versus $127.2 \pm 7.9$ pg/mg creatinine). A similar increment was evident in the excretion of the metabolite in cirrhosis ($1925.6 \pm 496.8$ versus $663.5 \pm 95.2$ pg/mg creatinine) as compared to that observed for the parent $iPF_{2\alpha}$-III. Thus, the increment in urinary $iPF_{2\alpha}$-III is likely to reflect its increased generation, rather than its decreased metabolism, in cirrhosis. Evidence for increased generation of isoprostanes in cirrhosis was confirmed by measurement of a second isoprostane, $iPF_{2\alpha}$-VI, in a subset of patients and controls. Urinary $iPF_{2\alpha}$-VI was also significantly elevated ($4.841 \pm 0.72$ versus $1.642 \pm 0.11$ pg/mg creatinine; $p < 0.001$) in cirrhosis. Levels of both isoprostanes were highly correlated ($r=0.9$; $p < 0.001$).

A third study involved assessment of isoprostane generation in patients with acute alcoholic hepatitis. Patients were admitted directly to the hepatology service from the emergency room. Not surprisingly, an even more marked increment in urinary excretion of both $iPF_{2\alpha}$-III and $iPF_{2\alpha}$-VI was demonstrated in patients with acute alcoholic hepatitis ($2205.07 \pm 408.2$ pg/mg creatinine; $p < 0.001$ and $20.405 \pm 4.772$ pg/mg creatinine; $p < 0.001$, respectively).

A fourth study addressed the effect of administration of vitamin C to patients with established liver disease. Given that $iPF_{2\alpha}$-III, but not $iPF_{2\alpha}$-VI, may be formed as a minor product of cyclooxygenase (COX) [9] we also assessed the effects of aspirin on these parameters. Patients were recruited from the hepatology and liver transplant clinics in the same manner mentioned for the preceding study. Five patients were studied in each group:

ALD, HCV, and combined disease. Baseline measurement of endogenous vitamin levels and urinary isoprostanes were obtained, as well as further demographic information including smoking history, prescribed drug intake, alcohol use, and prior or concurrent medical history. Patients were then instructed to take 2.5 grams of vitamin C per day for ten days. Upon return to the General Clinical Research Center (GCRC), repeat vitamin and isoprostane measurements were obtained. Patients then entered a ten-day "wash-out" period during which vitamin C intake was suspended, and following which they were studied again in an identical manner. At this point they were given 325 mg of aspirin (ASA). Urinary isoprostane measurement was repeated 24 hours after ASA ingestion. In this study we also compared measurement of TBARs, an *ex vivo* assay used to reflect ROS generation [10] with isoprostane production at identical time points. Plasma levels of vitamin C were $0.74 \pm 0.3$ mg/dL in ALD, $0.83 \pm 0.24$ mg/dL in HCV cirrhosis, $0.68 \pm 0.18$ mg/dL in combined disease, $0.36 \pm 0.16$ mg/dL in acute alcoholic hepatitis and $1.1 \pm 0.3$ mg/dL in healthy controls. Serum alpha tocopherol levels were $6.4 \pm 1.75$ mg/L for patients with ALD, $10.6 \pm 5.9$ mg/L for patients with HCV cirrhosis, $8.4 \pm 2.7$ mg/L in patients with combined disease, $4.15 \pm 2.2$ mg/dL in acute alcoholic hepatitis, and $11.3 \pm 2.1$ mg/L for healthy controls. Both urinary $iPF_{2\alpha}$-III and $iPF_{2\alpha}$-VI were elevated, as expected, at baseline in all patients ($763.8 \pm 139.3$ and $6.198 \pm 1.843$ pg/mg creatinine). Vitamin C ingestion suppressed urinary $iPF_{2?}$-III and $iPF_{2?}$-VI in patients with ALD and combined disease but had no significant effect in patients with HCV cirrhosis. For example, the delta decrease from baseline for $iPF_{2\alpha}$-III and $iPF_{2\alpha}$-VI was $396.04 \pm 117.4$ and $3.34 \pm 1.23$ pg/mg creatinine; $p < 0.001$, respectively, for patients with ALD; $226.5 \pm 139.3$ and $2.06 \pm 0.65$ pg/mg creatinine; $p < 0.05$, respectively, for patients with combined disease; and $90 \pm 100.2$ and $0.53 \pm 0.833$ pg/mg creatinine; $p < 0.2$, respectively, for patients with HCV cirrhosis.

Plasma levels of vitamin C were within the normal range at baseline for all patients ($1.78 \pm 1.3$ mg/dL). Levels rose following 10 days of vitamin C ingestion to $4.24 \pm 1.3$ mg/dL, and returned toward baseline values following discontinuation of the vitamin ($1.65 \pm 1.1$ mg/dL). Serum alpha tocopherol levels were $6.4 \pm 1.75$ mg/L for patients with ALD, $10.6 \pm 5.9$ mg/L for patients with hepatitis C cirrhosis (HCV), $8.4 \pm 2.7$ mg/L in patients with combined disease and $11.3 \pm 2.1$ mg/L for healthy controls.

Recently, there has been interest in the possibility that reactive oxygen indices (ROIs) might contribute to the evolution of ALD. It is recognized that chronic alcoholics frequently consume inadequate diets, which may be deficient in antioxidant vitamins [11]. Indeed, the antioxidant content of red wine has been suggested as an explanation for the association of cardiovascular benefit with this form of alcohol consumption [12], the so-called French Paradox. Rifici and Khachadurian [13] have recently reported that whereas alcohol enhances cell mediated lipoprotein oxidation, the same amount of red wine suppressed this effect. The polyphenols, carechin, and epicarechin appear to be the major contributors to the antioxidant properties of red wine [13].

The present study utilizes a novel approach to investigate the relationship between ROI generation *in vivo* and ALD. Isoeicosanoids are a family of free radical catalyzed products of arachidonic acid which are isomers of the conventional, enzymatically formed eicosanoids. These compounds, in contrast with conventional indices of oxidant stress, are chemically stable and may be measured specifically with GC/MS [14]. Attention has focused upon the $F_2$-isoprostanes, which circulate in plasma and are excreted in urine. They exist in 4 structure classes [15,16]. We have developed assays for members of two classes, $iPF_{2\alpha}$-III and $iPF_{2\alpha}$-VI, using GC/MS. Urinary excretion of these compounds are increased in a wide variety of syndromes of oxidant stress, including cigarette smoking [6], poisoning with acetaminophen and paraquat [5] and during reperfusion, following coronary ischemia [8,9]. Excretion is also increased in asymptomatic hypercholesterolemia and in patients with overt atherosclerosis [17,18]. We have recently immunolocalized the $iPF_{2\alpha}$-III to monocytes and smooth muscle cells in human atherosclerotic plaque [19].

We have previously reported that urinary $iPF_{2\alpha}$-III is elevated in patients with cirrhosis [20]. However, the majority of these patients (79%) had a history of antecedent viral hepatitis and a detailed history of alcohol consumption was not obtained. The present study extends these findings to elucidate the role of oxidant stress in ALD. Excretion of $iPF_{2\alpha}$-III is increased in patients with established cirrhosis and a history of antecedent alcohol abuse. Indeed, the increment in isoprostane excretion is more marked than that observed in cirrhotic patients with a history of hepatitis C. Furthermore, excretion of the isoprostane is increased in patients with acute alcoholic liver disease and, in a dose-dependent manner, by alcohol administration to healthy volunteers. In volunteers, alcohol administration resulted in a time-dependent increment in urinary $iPF_{2\alpha}$-III. Furthermore, both peak urinary excretion of the isoprostane and the area under the concentration-time curve were related to dose. Thus, oxidant stress is associated with alcohol consumption in volunteers, in patients with acute alcoholic hepatitis and in patients with cirrhosis and an antecedent history of alcohol abuse.

In addition to the increment in urinary $iPF_{2\alpha}$-III, we report that excretion of its 2,3-dinor-5,6-dihydro metabolite [21] is also increased in cirrhosis. This is the first report of formation of an isoprostane metabolite in a human disease. While the urinary levels of the metabolite are more abundant than those of the parent compound, excretion of both are increased in cirrhosis and correlate with each other. This provides evidence supportive of the concept that the increment in urinary $iPF_{2\alpha}$-III reflects an increase in its generation *in vivo*, rather than reduced oxidative metabolism due to impairment of hepatic function.

We have previously shown that $iPF_{2\alpha}$-III may be formed as a minor product of both COX isoforms [9,22]. However, evidence in healthy volunteers and in syndromes of COX activation suggest that these pathways contribute trivially, if at all, to urinary concentrations of the isoprostane [6,23]. Consistent with these observations, we report that vitamin C, but not aspirin, suppressed urinary $iPF_{2\alpha}$-III and TBARs in patients with alcoholic cirrhosis. These observations accord with the suppressive effects of vitamin E on the increment in urinary $iPF_{2\alpha}$-III in cirrhosis anteceded by viral hepatitis [20]. Furthermore, urinary excretion of $iPF_{2\alpha}$-VI, an isoprostane which is not formed by COX-dependent mechanisms [6,23] is also increased in patients with both acute alcoholic hepatitis and alcohol induced cirrhosis. These observations provide further evidence that ROI generation and lipid peroxidation are increased *in vivo* in patients with ALD.

The mechanisms which underlie the increase in oxidant stress in ALD are unclear. Although alcoholics often consume a diet deficient in antioxidant vitamins, our patients were stabilized on a standardized diet for two weeks prior to participation in the study. They also had abstained from alcohol for a minimum of 4 months prior to being studied. Although we did not make a formal assessment of all endogenous antioxidant defenses, their serum levels of vitamins C and E were normal.

These studies provide evidence for alcohol-induced free radical generation in healthy humans and in patients with acute and chronic ALD. Utilization of these noninvasive markers of lipid peroxidation is likely to elucidate the role of oxidant stress during the evolution of ALD. They may also be used to discriminate between the oxidant effects of various forms of alcohol and to titrate the dosage of antioxidant strategies designed to modify the evolution of this disease.

## References

1.    Lieber CS, DeCarli LM. Hepatic microsomal ethanol-oxidizing system. In vitro characteristics and adaptive properties in vivo. J Biol Chem 1970;245:2505-12.
2.    Tsukamoto H. Oxidative stress, antioxidants, and alcoholic liver fibrogenesis. Alcohol 1993;10:465-67.
3.    Morrow JD, Hill KE, Burk RF, Nammour TM, Badr KF, Roberts LJ 2d. A series of prostaglandin F2-like compounds are produced in vivo in humans by a non-cyclooxygenase, free radical-catalyzed mechanism. Proc Nat Acad Sci USA 1990;87: 9383-87.
4.    Morrow JD, Minton TA, Mukundan CR, et al. Free radical-induced generation of isoprostanes in vivo. Evidence for the formation of D-ring and E-ring isoprostanes. J Biol Chem 1994;269(6):4317-26.
5.    Delanty N, Reilly MP, Praticó D, Fitzgerald DJ, Lawson JA, FitzGerald, GA. 8-epi PGF2α specific analysis of an isoeicosanoid as an index of oxidant stress. Br J Clin Pharm 1996; 42:15-19.
6.    Reilly M, Delanty N, Lawson JA, FitzGerald GA. Modulation of oxidant stress in vivo in chronic cigarette smokers. Circulation 1996;94:19-25.
7.    Delanty N, Reilly MP, Praticó D, et al. 8-epi PGF$_{2\alpha}$ generation during coronary reperfusion A potential quantitative marker of oxidant stress *in vivo*. Circulation 1997;95: 2492-99.
8.    Reilly M, Delanty N, Roy L, O'Callaghan P, Crean P, FitzGerald GA. Increased generation of the F$_2$ isoprostanes, IPF$_{2\alpha}$-I and 8-epi PGF$_{2\alpha}$ in acute coronary angioplasty: Evidence for oxidant stress during coronary reperfusion in humans. Circulation 1997;96: 3314-20.
9.    Pratico D, Lawson JA, FitzGerald GA. Cyclooxygenase dependent formation of 8-epi PGF$_{2\alpha}$ in human platelets. J Biol Chem 1995;270:9800-9808.
10.   Smith CV, Anderson RE. Methods for determination of lipid peroxidation in biological samples. Free Rad Biol Med 1987;3:341-44.
11.   Leo MA, Rosman AS, Lieber CS, Differential depletion of carotenoids and tocopherol in

liver disease. Hepatology 1993;17:977-86.

12.     Frankel EN, Kanner J, German JB, Parks E, Kinsella JE. Inhibition of oxidation of human low-density lipoprotein by phenolic substances in red wine. Lancet 1993;341:454-457.

13.     Rifici VA, Khachadurian AK. Polyphenols found in red wine inhibit cell mediated lipoprotein oxidation. J Invest Med 1998;46(suppl):2907A.

14.     Patrono C, FitzGerald GA. Isoprostanes: Potential markers of oxidant stress in atherothrombotic disease. Arterio Throm Vasc Biol (Brief Review) 1997;17:2309-15.

15.     Rokach J, Khanapure S.P, Hwang S-W, Adiyaman M, Lawson JA, FitzGerald GA. Nomenclature of isoprostanes: A proposal. Prostaglandins 1997;54:853-73.

16.     Waugh RJ, Murphy RC. Mass spectrometric analysis of four regioisomers of $F_2$-isoprostanes formed by free radical oxidation of arachidonic acid. J Am Soc Mass Spectrom 1996;7:490-99.

17.     Reilly M, Praticó D, Delanty N, et al. Increased generation of distinct $F_2$ isoprostanes in hypercholesterolemia. Circulation 1998;98(25):2822-28.

18.     Davi G, Alessandrini P, Mezzetti A, et al. *In vivo* formation of 8-epi-prostaglandin $F_{2\alpha}$ is increased in hypercholesterolemia. Arterioscler Thromb Vasc Biol 1997;17:3230-35.

19.     Pratico D, Juliano J, Mauriello A, et al. Localization of distinct $F_2$ isoprostanes in human atherosclerotic lesions. J Clin Invest 1997;100:2028-34.

20.     Iuliano L, Pratico D, Ferro D, et al. Enhanced lipid peroxidation in patients with hepatic cirrhosis. J Invest Med 1998;46:51-57.

21.     Roberts LJ, II, Moore KP, Zackert WE, Oates JA, Morrow JD. Identification of the major urinary metabolite of the $F_2$-isoprostane 8-iso-prostaglandin $F_{2\alpha}$ in humans. J Biol Chem 1996;271:20617-20.

22.     Pratico D, FitzGerald GA. Generation of 8-epi $PGF_{2\alpha}$ by human monocytes: Discrimination production by reactive oxygen species and PG G/H S-2. J Biol Chem 1996; 271:8919-24.

23.     Pratico D, Barry OP, Lawson JA, et al. $IPF_{2\alpha}$-I: An index of lipid peroxidation in humans. Proc Natl Acad Sci (USA) 1998;95:3449-54.

ANTIATHEROGENIC EFFECTS OF NONALCOHOLIC INGREDIENTS IN ALCOHOLIC BEVERAGES

Hiroshige Itakura, Kazuo Kondo, and Akiyo Matsumoto

## Introduction

Oxidative modification of low density lipoprotein (LDL) by free radicals may play a central role in the development of atherosclerosis [1]. Increased intake of antioxidants has been suggested in epidemiological studies to be associated with decreased risk of coronary heart disease [2-5]. Phenolics are one of the major groups of nonessential dietary components; however, both essential and nonessential dietary antioxidants are thought to be beneficial for prevention of atherosclerosis and cancer. Wine and beer contain many kinds of polyphenols. Several phenolic compounds have been shown to have antioxidant properties *in vitro*, inhibiting the oxidative modification of LDL and inhibiting platelet aggregation [6,7]. However it is necessary to demonstrate antioxidant effects *in vivo* after ingestion of polyphenol-rich alcoholic beverages.

## Inhibition of Oxidation of LDL with Red Wine

Moderate intake of alcoholic beverages has been shown to increase high density lipoprotein (HDL) cholesterol in plasma and to reduce thrombotic tendencies. To distinguish between the antioxidant properties of red wine and other alcoholic beverages without polyphenol components, we studied the effects of red wine compared with vodka [8]. Ten male volunteers (33-57 years old) drank vodka (40% ethanol) (washout period) and then red wine (Chateau Lagrange, 1989) (experimental period), corresponding to a dose of 0.8 g/kg ethanol per day for 14 days. All subjects received the same standard diet (supplied by Taihei Co., Tokyo) to control their caloric and nutritional intake, and they abstained from drinking tea, coffee, and other such substances to minimize the intake of phenolic substances other than those derived from red wine throughout the study period. Fasting venous blood samples were taken at days -14, 0, and +14. Plasma LDL was prepared by ultra centrifugation (d 1.006-1,063 g/ml) and oxidizability of LDL was investigated by measuring conjugated diens formed with 2,2'-azobis (4-methoxy-2,4-dimethylvaleronitrite; V-70).

The results of LDL oxidation experiments are shown in Figure 1. The induction period or lag phase was significantly longer at day 14 (54.7[SE 2.6] min) than at day 0

73

*R. Paoletti et al. (eds.), Moderate Alcohol Consumption and Cardiovascular Disease, 73–79.*
© 2000 *Kluwer Academic Publishers and Fondazione Giovanni Lorenzini. Printed in the Netherlands.*

(49.1 [SE 2.2] min). There was no difference in LDL oxidation between day -14 and day 0. These results suggest that continuous intake of red wine, but not of ethanol, may inhibit LDL oxidation *in vivo*. Serum concentrations of vitamin E, β-carotene, and vitamin C did not change during the study period. Serum total cholesterol (TC) levels did not change during the washout period, but during the experimental period serum TC level decreased significantly ($p < 0.05$) from $206 \pm 9.2$ mg/dl to $191 \pm 9.2$ mg/dl. Serum free cholesterol, triglyceride (TG), HDL-cholesterol, phospholipids, free fatty acid, and apolipoproteins (A1, A2, B, C2, C3, E) levels remained unchanged throughout the study period (Table 1). Serum Lp(a) level decreased after intake of red wine. During the washout period serum Lp(a) level did not change; on the other hand, serum Lp(a) level decreased significantly ($p < 0.01$) from 24.1 mg/dl to 22.0 mg/dl during the experimental period. Significant reductions of Lp(a) were observed in subjects with a level of Lp(a) higher than 30 mg/dl (Figure 2). Sharpe et al. have reported that red wine, 200 ml per day for 10 days, reduced Lp(a) significantly ($p < 0.001$) and increased membrane fluidity ($p < 0.01$) [9]. Lp(a) is recognized as an independent risk factor for atherosclerosis; the reduction of serum level of Lp(a) induced by regular and long-term consumption of red wine may thus be beneficial for prevention of atherosclerotic diseases.

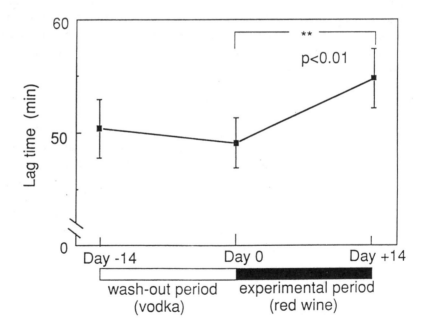

Figure 1. Effect of red wine consumption on LDL oxidation in volunteers. N=10. Values are means (SE). Paired t test.

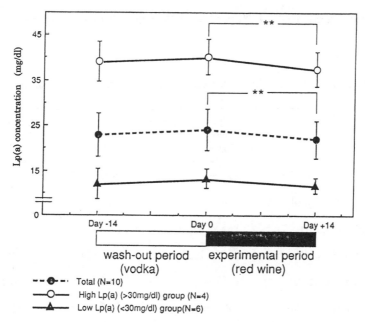

Figure 2. Effect of red wine consumption on serum Lp(a) levels in volunteers. N=10, Values are means (SE). Paired t test.

The lag time of LDL oxidation was observed to be correlated with the concentration of total phenolic substances in red wine (r=0.6752, p < 0.001) (Figure 3). Many kinds of nonalcoholic substances are detected in red wine and phenolic substances may have a central role in the inhibition of oxidation of LDL, but further studies may be needed to explain the associated effect of Lp(a) reduction.

## Red Wine Improves Flow-Mediated Vasodilatation

The impairment of vascular endothelial function is thought to be an important factor in the development of atherosclerosis. Endothelial dysfunction may cause the impairment of endothelium-derived relaxing factor (EDRF) release from endothelial cells. Certain wines, grape juices, and grape skin extracts relaxed precontracted smooth muscle of intact rat aortic rings, an effect reversed by the nitric oxide (NO) synthase inhibitor, N-methyl-L-arginine acetate, a competitive inhibitor of the synthesis of the EDRF [10,11]; the same type of vasorelaxation was also observed by using human coronary arteries *in vitro* [12]. The effects of ingesting purple grape juice on endothelial function and LDL susceptibility to oxidation in patients with coronary artery disease have been reported [13]. Flow-mediated vasodilatation (FMD) was measured using high-resolution brachial artery ultrasonography. At baseline, FMD was impaired (2.2 ± 2.9%). After ingestion of grape juice, FMD increased to 6.4 ± 4.7% (p=0.003). Polyphenols in purple grape juice may have improved endothelium-dependent vasodilatation and increased LDL oxidation lag time by 34.5%.

Table 1. Effect of Red Wine Consumption on Risk Factors for Atherosclerosis

|  | Washout period | Experimental period | |
| --- | --- | --- | --- |
|  | Day -14 | Day 0 | Day +14 |
| Total cholesterol (mg/dl) | 211 ± 11.4 | 206 ± 9.2 | 191 ± 9.2* |
| Free cholesterol (mg/dl) | 54 ± 3.1 | 56 ± 4.6 | 50 ± 3.2 |
| Triglycerides (mg/dl) | 155 ± 37.2 | 263 ± 113.2 | 184 ± 52.0 |
| Phospholipids (mg/dl) | 248 ± 16.3 | 243 ± 20.0 | 240 ± 14.9 |
| Free fatty acids (mg/dl) | 0.53 ± 0.1 | 0.65 ± 0.1 | 0.59 ± 0.1 |
| HDL cholesterol (mg/dl) | 58.0 ± 3.4 | 55.0 ± 4.6 | 55.2 ± 4.1 |
| Apolipoproteins (mg/dl) |  |  |  |
| A-1 | 162 ± 8.7 | 163 ± 12.0 | 157 ± 4.1 |
| A-2 | 39 ± 2.0 | 42 ± 4.5 | 41 ± 2.8 |
| B | 107 ± 9.2 | 122 ± 22.4 | 103 ± 12.3 |
| C-2 | 4.6 ± 0.6 | 4.7 ± 0.7 | 4.7 ± 0.6 |
| C-3 | 16 ± 2.0 | 16 ± 2.7 | 16 ± 2.3 |
| E | 4.6 ± 0.4 | 5.0 ± 0.9 | 4.3 ± 0.6 |

Values are mean ± SE; *: $p < 0.05$ versus Day 0.

To elucidate whether acute intake of red wine improves macrovascular endothelial function in men, seven healthy men were each scheduled to drink 500 ml water, Japanese vodka (Schochu) (0.8 g/kg ethanol), red wine (Chateau Beychevell, 0.8 g/kg ethanol), and red wine without alcohol within a 30-minute period [14]. The brachial artery diameter was measured noninvasively using a 7.5 MHz ultrasound probe at rest and during reactive hyperemia, which causes endothelium-dependent vasodilatation. Improvement of flow-mediated diameter increase was observed 120 minutes after red wine intake (8.1 ± 0.5% versus 6.9 ± 0.7%, $p < 0.05$). The improvement was also observed 30 minutes after intake of red wine without alcohol (10.3 ± 1.3% versus 6.7 ± 0.6%, $p < 0.01$). No improvement was observed after intake of water or Japanese vodka. These results indicate that nonalcoholic constituents of red wine improve endothelium-dependent vasodilatation.

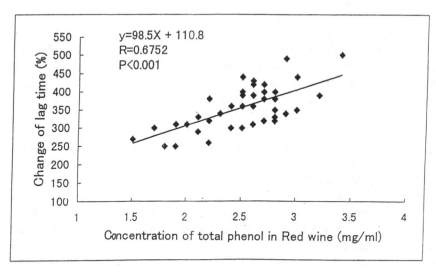

Figure 3. Correlation between the concentration of total phenol in red wine and change of the lag time of LDL oxidation.

## Red Wine Polyphenols Inhibit Proliferation of Vascular Smooth Muscle Cells

Vascular smooth muscle cell (VSMC) proliferation is known to play an important role in the progression of atherosclerotic lesions. The effects of red wine polyphenols on VSMC proliferation have been studied [15]. Total polyphenolic fraction was extracted from red wine by adsorption chromatography and this fraction was further separated into six fractions by successive column chromatography. Treatment with red wine polyphenolic fraction showed a potent inhibitory effect on the proliferation and DNA synthesis of cultured rat aortic smooth muscle cells from concentrations as low as 1 µg/ml. In contrast, this fraction did not significantly inhibit the proliferation and DNA synthesis of vascular endothelial cells. The average molecular weights of red wine polyphenolic fraction were distributed approximately between 200-400 and 1600-2000. The lower molecular weight fractions contain various polyphenolic monomer components, such as anthocyanidine, resveratrol, catechins, and flavonoids and the highest fraction contained almost 100% proanthocyanidins. It is noteworthy that polyphenol fractions of different molecular weight showed similar potent antiproliferative effects on VSMC. Duthie et al. measured the plasma concentration of polyphenolic monomers after the intake of red wine and reported that the intake of 100 ml red wine resulted in an increase in plasma concentration of 2.5 µg/ml [16]. The antiproliferative effects on VSMC of red wine polyphenols may be associated with the downregulation of cyclin A gene expression through the inhibition of transcription factor expression.

## Cardioprotective Effects of Red Wine

Red wine has also been reported to increase coronary flow-velocity reserve [17]. Coronary flow-velocity reserve (CFVR) is known to be an indicator of the functional significance of ischemic heart disease. Epicardial coronary blood flow velocity was measured noninvasively by transthoracic color doppler echocardiography (TTDE). The effects of red wine on coronary microcirculation *in vivo* by noninvasive assessment by CFVR with TTDE were investigated and compared with the effects of white wine and vodka. A significant increase in CFVR was observed after intake of red wine (from $3.2 \pm 0.7$ to $4.2 \pm 1.2$, p=0.0016), but not after intake of white wine or vodka. It was speculated that some polyphenols in red wine might have vasorelaxing effects on coronary microvessels during hyperemia. The potential cardioprotective effects of resveratrol were observed in the face of ischemia reperfusion injury [18]. In experiments on isolated perfused working rat hearts, infarct size was markedly reduced in the resveratrol group when compared to the control group. This study suggests that the red wine antioxidant resveratrol possesses cardioprotective effects.

## Conclusion

Red wine contains phenolic compounds such as proanthocyanidins, anthocyanidins, resveratrol, cathechins, and flavonoids. Intake of red wine reduces the susceptibility of LDL to oxidation and its potent antioxidant properties may be derived from the nonalcoholic components of red wine. Prevention of platelet aggregation, improvement of endothelial function, and cardioprotective effects have been observed by short-term ingestion of red wine. The phenolic compounds in alcoholic beverages, independent of alcohol content, may be beneficial for prevention of atherosclerosis.

## References

1.    Steinberg D, Pathasarathy S, Carew TE, Khoo JC, Witztum JL. Modifications of low-density lipoprotein that increase its atherogenesity. N Engl J Med 1989;320:915-24.
2.    Hertog MGL, Feskens EJM, Hollman PCH, Katan MB, Kromhout D. Dietary antioxidant flavonoids and risk of coronary heart disease: The Zutphen Elderly Study. Lancet 1993; 342:1007-11.
3.    Street DA, Comstock GW, Salkeld RM, et al. A population-based case-control study of the association of serum antioxidants and myocardial infarction. Am J Epidemiol 1991; 134:719-20.
4.    Gey KF, Moser UK, Jordan P, et al. Increased risk of cardiovascular disease at suboptimal plasma concentrations of essential antioxidants: An epidemiological update with special attention to carotene and vitamin C. Am J Clin Nutr 1993;57(Suppl.):787S-97S.
5.    Knekt P, Järvinen R, Reunanen A, Maatela J. Flavonoid intake and coronary mortality in

Finland: A cohort study. BMJ 1996;312:478-81.

6. Frankel EN, Kanner J, German JB, Parks E, Kinsella JE. Inhibition of oxidation of low-density lipoprotein by phenolic substances in red wine. Lancet 1993;341:454-57.

7. Pace-Asciak CR, Hahn S, Diamandis EP, Soleas G, Goldberg DM. The red wine phenolics trans-resveratrol and quercetin block human platelet aggregation and eicosanoid synthesis: Implications for protection against coronary heart disease. Clin Chim Acta 1995;235: 207-19.

8. Kondo K, Matsumoto A, Kurata H, et al. Inhibition of oxidation of low-density lipoprotein with red wine. Lancet 1994;344:1152.

9. Sharpe PC, McGrath LT, McClean E, Young IS, Archbold GP. Effect of red wine consumption on lipoprotein (a) and other risk factors for atherosclerosis. QJM 1995;88: 101-8.

10. Fitzpatrick DF, Hirschfield SL, Coffey RG. Endothelium-dependent vasorelaxing activity of wine and other grape products. Am J Physiol 1993;265:h774-78.

11. Cishek MB, Galloway MT, Karim M, German JB, Kappagoda CT. Effect of red wine on endothelium-dependent relaxation in rabbits. Clin Sci 1997;93:507-11.

12. Fleech M, Schwarz A, Bohm M. Effects of red and white wine on endothelium-dependent vasorelaxation of rat aorta and human coronary arteries. Am J Physiol 1998;275:h1183-90.

13. Stein JH, Keevil JG, Wiebe DA, Aeschlimann S, Folte JD. Purple grape juice improves endothelial function and reduces the susceptibility of LDL cholesterol to oxidation in patients with coronary artery disease. Circulation 1999;100:1050-55.

14. Hashimoto M, Kim S, Eto M, et al. Acute intake of red wine improves flow-mediated vasodilatation of the brachial artery in men. Unpublished data.

15. Iijima K, Yoshizumi M, Hashimoto M, et al. Red wine polyphenols inhibit proliferation of vascular smooth muscle cells and downregulate expression of cyclin A gene. In preparation.

16. Duthie GG, Pedersen MW, Gardner PT, et al. The effect of whisky and wine consumption on total phenol content and antioxidant capacity of plasma from healthy volunteers. Eur J Clin Nutr 1998;52:733-36.

17. Shimada K., Watanabe H, Hosoda K, Takeuchi K, Yoshikawa J. Effect of red wine on coronary flow-velocity reserve. Lancet 1999;354:1002.

18. Ray PS, Maulik G, Cordis GA, Bertelle AAE, Bertelli A, Das DK. The red wine antioxidant resveratrol protects isolated rat hearts from ischemia reperfusion injury. Free Radic Biol Med 1999;27:160-69.

# ALCOHOL INTAKE, DRINKING HABITS, AND CORONARY HEART DISEASE

Kari Poikolainen

## Introduction

"Doctor, is alcohol good for my heart?" This seems to be a frequently asked question when patients and doctors meet. This paper reviews the epidemiologic evidence on the relation between alcohol and coronary heart disease (CHD), discusses the interpretation of the findings, and suggests an approach to advising patients. Strong evidence shows that CHD risk is lowest among moderate drinkers and highest among heavy drinkers. The optimal level for a healthy adult person cannot be determined exactly but it may be around one to three drinks a day. Drinking small amounts almost every day seems to protect the individual from CHD better than less frequent moderate drinking. Individualized advice should weigh the decrease in CHD risk against the risk of alcohol dependence and alcohol-related diseases.

## What Has Been Found?

Several studies have found that the risk of CHD is lower among moderate drinkers than among abstainers [1]. For example, the American Cancer Society Study found that mortality from CHD was, compared with nondrinkers, 10%-30% lower among alcohol-consuming men with no pre-existing CHD, and 30%-40% lower among men with pre-existing CHD. The respective figures for women were 10%-20% and 30%-40% [2].

## Is the Relation Causal?

Causal conclusions are commonly based on criteria suggested by Sir Austin Bradford Hill [3]. The evidence on the relation between alcohol intake and CHD seems to meet most of the accepted criteria well.

The cause precedes the effect in case-control studies that have been based on only incident cases and in follow-up studies where the cohort members have been initially free of CHD. The relation has been observed in both ecological, case-control, and follow-up studies.

The relation has been found in many populations. These include as diverse countries as Australia [4], Finland [5], Italy [6,7], Japan [8], New Zealand [9], Scotland [10], Sweden

81

*R. Paoletti et al. (eds.), Moderate Alcohol Consumption and Cardiovascular Disease,* 81–87.
© 2000 *Kluwer Academic Publishers and Fondazione Giovanni Lorenzini. Printed in the Netherlands.*

[11] and in the United States from Boston [12] to California [13] and to Japanese Americans living in Hawaii [14].

Most studies have focused on middle-aged men. However, the decrease in CHD risk has also been observed in older men and women [15-18] and in premenopausal women [19].

Not all studies have found a difference between abstainers and moderate drinkers in CHD risk or in all-cause death risk [20,21]. Differences are not likely to be found if healthy subjects are followed up for a short time only or if the subjects are young. In longer follow ups differences tend to emerge. For example, in the 25-year follow up of Swedish male conscripts the results suggest a negative trend between alcohol intake and the risk of myocardial infarction albeit nonsignificantly [11].

The higher mortality among nondrinkers is not only due to the selection of ex-drinkers or sick subjects into the group of abstainers. The CHD risk has been found to be higher among lifelong abstainers than among light drinkers even after controlling for smoking and several other factors [14,18,22,23]. The relation does not seem to be due to confounding, since almost all known confounders have been controlled for. An unknown confounder, if there were one, had to be very strong and unevenly distributed between moderate drinkers and abstainers to be able to explain the relation.

The association is rather strong. The estimates from various studies suggest that risk of CHD is 20%-60% lower among moderate drinkers than among abstainers. Some, but not all, studies suggest a negative linear dose-response relationship [12-14,23].

The epidemiologic evidence is in line with studies on atherosclerosis. Alcohol administration to monkeys has been found to decrease cholesterol-induced atherosclerosis in the coronary arteries and in the aorta [24]. Human angiographic studies have shown that abstainers have more atherosclerotic lesions than moderate drinkers [25]. Likewise, incident carotic atherosclerosis has been found to be less common among moderate drinkers (1-50 g of alcohol a day) than among irregular drinkers [26].

Two biologic effects of alcohol seem to explain the decrease of CHD risk in drinkers: increase in high-density lipoprotein cholesterol (HDL) and decrease in blood clotting tendency. Many studies have shown that alcohol increases HDL levels [27-31]. The relative increase in subfractions $HDL_2$ and $HDL_3$ seem to vary depending on gender, drinking habits, and exercise patterns of the subjects studied. Both $HDL_2$ and $HDL_3$ associate with myocardial infarction, and both subfractions seem to have an important role in providing protection from atherosclerosis and CHD [12,32].

There is less evidence on the positive effects of alcohol on blood clotting activity and insulin resistance. Cross-sectional population studies have found lower insulin levels among drinkers than abstainers [33-34]. Randomized studies have found favorable changes in thrombolysis and coagulation [35-36]. That these effects may be of clinical importance is suggested by lower occurrence of acute coronary attacks among persons having consumed alcohol within the preceding 24 hours than among abstainers [37].

In contrast to moderate drinkers, heavy drinkers seem to have higher CHD risk than abstainers. The Chicago Gas Company Study found that the risk of CHD death was 2.2-fold increased risk among problem drinkers compared with all other men [38]. In the British Regional Heart Study, an intake of 5 drinks or more a day was found to increase the risk of sudden cardiac death [39]. In Finland, significantly increased risk of CHD death has been found in relation to heavy drinking [40], frequency of intoxication and of hangover [41], and drinking six or more beers on one occasion [42].

Overall, epidemiologic studies thus suggest that the relation between alcohol and CHD is curvilinear, U-shaped, or J-shaped. The shape observed may depend on the amount of intake and drinking patterns of subjects taking part in various studies. An Australian case-control study illustrates the importance of drinking patterns. CHD (acute myocardial infarction and sudden coronary death) was studied in over 11,000 cases and 6,000 controls [4]. Age, blood pressure, and history of coronary heart disease were controlled for. The findings suggest that moderate and frequent drinking decreases the risk of CHD while heavy drinking increases the risk, perhaps independent of the frequency of drinking. The lowest CHD risk was found at the level of 10-20 g of alcohol per day on 5-6 days a week among both men and women (odds ratio (OR)=0.4). The highest risks of CHD risk were found among men consuming 90 g or more a day 1-2 days a week (OR=2.6) or daily (OR=2.4) and among women consuming 50 g or more a day 1-2 days a week (OR=1.6).

The curvilinear relation seems to be explained by the fact that alcohol has, in addition to the beneficial biologic effects, also harmful effects. Alcohol may increase blood pressure [43]. In one randomized trial, an average intake of 25 g a day was found to increase blood pressure among some but not all normotensive men [29]. The pressor effect seems to be fully reversible, since former heavy drinkers aged 20-44 years have been found to have blood pressures similar to lifelong abstainers [44]. There seems to be a threshold effect. The threshold has been estimated to be, on the average, from 30 to 60 g of alcohol a day [45].

Heavy drinking seems to accelerate atherosclerosis. Angiographic studies have shown that binge drinkers have more stenosis in their coronary arteries than individuals that consumed the same total amount of alcohol in more frequent but smaller amounts [46]. Incident carotic atherosclerosis has been found to be more common among heavy drinkers with an intake of 100 g of alcohol or more a day than among irregular drinkers [26].

Clinical observations suggest that heavy drinking increases the risk of disturbances of the rhythm of the heart [43]. Heavy drinking may also impair the activity of autonomic nervous system and decrease the complexity of heart rate dynamics [47-48].

The negative and positive effects of alcohol go together. In a randomized trial among healthy, moderately drinking males aged 20-45 years, alcohol restriction decreased both blood pressure and HDL-level. Decrease in the latter could not be compensated by a vigorous exercise program [30]. The net effect of alcohol mediated by changes in cholesterol metabolism and blood pressure on mortality and CHD is positive at the moderate intake level. Controlling for hypertension or blood pressure has not had any notable influence on the difference in CHD risk between abstainers and moderate drinkers when compared with unadjusted figures [19,20,22,23]. At least 50% of the protective effect of alcohol on CHD seems to be mediated by increases in HDL [49].

## From Research into Practice

The evidence for both beneficial and harmful effects of alcohol intake on CHD risk seems to be approximately as strong as the evidence for the relation between alcohol and liver cirrhosis or alcohol and aerodigestive cancer. Should this influence advising patients? Or should we wait for stronger evidence, obtained only by randomized clinical trials? Although such trials would be useful to determine the optimal dose of alcohol and to identify possible side effects of moderate intake, it does not seem likely that these trials will ever be done. If so, it seems better to base advice on available evidence than to ignore the evidence.

In advising individual patients, the best course of action might be to compare carefully the potential benefits and costs of alcohol intake. Protection from CHD by alcohol seems to be especially beneficial for men, for the old and middle-aged, for patients with CHD, and for healthy individuals with a family history of CHD. On the other hand, abstaining might be the healthiest choice for many patients with certain diseases, such as depression, hypertension, liver cirrhosis, or peptic ulcer, when these are alcohol-related. Risk of alcohol dependence should also be considered.

Familial alcoholism increases the risk of alcoholism 3 to 4-fold among the offspring compared with persons without alcoholism in the family [50]. Persons suffering from major depression, anxiety disorder, antisocial disorder, or conduct disorder are also at increased risk. Future alcoholics tend to be heavy drinkers already in adolescence. Of all patients aged 18-62 years with the diagnosis of alcohol dependence, 97% had started drinking alcoholic beverages before the age of 18 years [51]. To my knowledge there are only a few studies that help us to estimate the potential risk of alcoholism among moderate drinkers. Among Swedish male conscripts aged 18-21 years and reporting abstinence from alcohol at the baseline examination, the risk of hospital inpatient admission for alcoholism over a follow up of 15 years was lower (RR=0.5; 95% CI 0.3-0.7) than among men reporting an intake of 1-100 g of alcohol a week [52]. Unfortunately, we do not know whether the weekly intake was consumed at one sitting or spread evenly over the whole week. In a cohort of adult Californians, both men and women changing from abstinence to moderate drinking had nonsignificantly lower age-adjusted all-cause mortality than adults who continued to abstain [53]. Research seems to suggest that moderate drinking starting in early twenties or later may not be particularly risky, if the subject has no psychiatric disorder or a history of familial alcoholism.

In the assessment of risks and benefits, monitoring of blood pressure and other risk factors seems to be advisable. Drinkers should know what moderation means, watch for any harmful effects of alcohol, and avoid intoxication. Unfortunately, we cannot say which is the best, most optimal moderate intake. The self-reports of alcohol intake tend to be underestimates of actual consumption. The average percentage of underestimation varies greatly (from 29% to 83%) between studies [54]. Although we know that there is some underestimation, it is difficult to correct for it because the degree of underestimation varies between studies and between individuals. However, a conservative estimate, based on the face value of the available evidence, suggests that the optimal level for a healthy adult man may be around one to three drinks a day, and for a woman slightly less, perhaps one to two drinks a day. This pertains both to the risk of CHD and all-cause mortality.

## References

1.    Rimm EB, Klatsky A, Grobbee D, Stampfer MJ. Review of moderate alcohol consumption and reduced risk of coronary heart disease: Is the effect due to beer, wine, or spirits? BMJ 1996;312:731-36.

2.    Thun MJ, Peto R, Lopez AD, Monaco JH, Henley SJ, Heath CW, Doll R. Alcohol consumption and mortality among middle-aged and elderly U.S. citizens. N Engl J Med 1997;337:1705-14.

3.    Hill AB. The environment and disease: Association or causation? Proc Roy Soc Med 1965;58:295-300.

4.    McElduff P, Dobson A. How much alcohol and how often? Population based case-control study of alcohol consumption and risk of a major coronary event. BMJ 1997;314:1159-64.

5.    Paunio M, Virtamo J, Gref C-G, Heinonen OP. Serum high density lipoprotein cholesterol, alcohol, and coronary mortality in male smokers. BMJ 1996;312:1200-1203.

6.    Rabajoli F, Arneodo D, Balzola F, Leo L, Vineis P. Moderate alcohol intake and risk of myocardial infarction among non-smokers. Eur J Public Health 1996;6:227-30.

7.    Tavani A, La Vecchia C, Negri E, D'Avanzo B, Franzosi M, Tognoni G. Alcohol intake and risk of myocardial infarction in Italian men. J Epidemiol Biostat 1996;1:31-39.

8.    Kitamura A, Iso H, Sankai T. Alcohol intake and premature coronary heart disease in urban Japanese men. Am J Epidemiol 1998;147:59-65.

9.    Jackson R, Scragg R, Beaglehole R. Alcohol consumption and risk of coronary heart disease. BMJ 1991;303:211-16.

10.   Woodward M, Tunstall-Pedoe H. Alcohol consumption, diet, coronary risk factors, and prevalent coronary heart disease in men and women in the Scottish heart health study. J Epidemiol Community Health 1995;49:354-62.

11.   Romelsjö A, Leifman A. Association between alcohol consumption and mortality, myocardial infarction, and stroke in 25 year follow up of 49 618 young Swedish men. BMJ 1999;319:821-22.

12.   Gaziano JM, Buring JE, Breslow JL, Goldhaber SZ, Rosner B, VanDenburgh M, Willett W, Hennekens CH. Moderate alcohol intake, increased levels of high density lipoprotein and its subfractions, and decreased risk of myocardial infarction. N Engl J Med 1993;329:1829-34.

13.   Klatsky AL, Friedman GD, Siegelaub AB. Alcohol consumption before myocardial infarction: results from the Kaiser-Permanente epidemiologic study of myocardial infarction. Ann Intern Med 1974;81:294-301.

14.   Yano K, Rhoads GG, Kagan A. Coffee, alcohol and risk of coronary heart disease among Japanese men living in Hawaii. N Engl J Med 1977;297:405-9.

15.   Kono S, Ikeda M, Ogata M, Tokudome S, Nishizumi M, Kuratsune M. The relationship between alcohol and mortality among Japanese physicians. Int J Epidemiol 1983;12:437-41.

16.   Colditz GA, Branch LG, Lipnick RJ, et al. Moderate alcohol and decreased cardiovascular mortality in an elderly cohort. Am Heart J 1985;109:886-89.

17.   Scherr PA, LaCroix AZ, Wallace RB, et al. Light to moderate alcohol consumption and

mortality in the elderly. J Am Geriatr Soc 1992;40:651-57.

18.    de Labry LO, Glynn RJ, Levenson MR, Hermos JA, LoCastro JS, Vokonas PS. Alcohol consumption and mortality in an American male population: recovering the U-shaped curve. J Stud Alcohol 1992;53:25-32.

19.    Stampfer MJ, Colditz GA, Willett WC, Speizer FE, Hennekens CH. A prospective study of moderate alcohol consumption and the risk of coronary disease and stroke in women. New Engl J Med 1988;319:267-73.

20.    Shaper AG, Wannamethee G, Walker M. Alcohol and mortality in British men: explaining the U-shaped curve. Lancet 1988;2:1267-73.

21.    Rehm J, Sempos CT. Alcohol consumption and all-cause mortality. Addiction 1995;90: 471-80.

22.    Klatsky AL, Armstrong MA, Friedman GD. Relations of alcoholic beverage use to subsequent coronary artery disease hospitalization. Am J Cardiol 1986;58:710-14.

23.    Rimm EB, Giovannucci EL, Willett WC, et al. Prospective study of alcohol consumption and risk of coronary disease in men. Lancet 1991;338:464-68.

24.    Rudel LL, Leathers CW, Bond MG, Bullock BC. Dietary ethanol-induced modifications in hyperlipoproteinemia and atherosclerosis in nonhuman primates [Macaca nemestrina]. Arteriosclerosis 1981;1:144-55.

25.    Barboriak JJ, Rimm AA, Anderson AJ, Schmidhoffer M, Tristani FE. Coronary artery occlusion and alcohol intake. Br Heart J 1977;39:289-93.

26.    Kiechl S, Willeit J, Rungger G, Egger G, Oberhollezer F, Bonora E. Alcohol consumption and atherosclerosis: What is the relation? Prospective results from the Bruneck Study. Stroke 1998;20:900-907.

27.    Castelli WP, Doyle JT, Gordon T, et al. Alcohol and blood lipids - the co-operative lipoprotein phenotyping study. Lancet 1977;ii:153-55.

28.    Välimäki M, Nikkilä EA, Taskinen M-R, Ylikahri R. Rapid decrease in high density lipoprotein subfractions and postheparin plasma lipase activities after cessation of chronic alcohol intake. Atherosclerosis 1986;59:147-53.

29.    Puddey IB, Beilin LJ, Vandongen R, Rouse IL, Rogers P. Evidence for a direct effect of alcohol consumption on blood pressure in normotensive men: a randomized controlled trial. Hypertension 1985;7:707-13.

30.    Cox KL, Puddey IB, Morton AR, Beilin LJ, Vandongen R, Masarei JRL. The combined effects of aerobic exercise and alcohol restriction on blood pressure and serum lipids: A two-way factorial study in sedentary men. J Hypertension 1993;11: 191-201.

31.    Hartung GH, Lawrence SJ, Reeves RS, Foreyt JP. Effect of alcohol and exercise on postprandial lipemia and triglyceride clearance in men. Atherosclerosis 1993;100:33-40.

32.    Stampfer MJ, Sacks FM, Salvini S, Willett WC, Hennekens CH. A prospective study of cholesterol, apolipoproteins, and the risk of myocardial infarction. N Engl J Med 1991;325: 373-81.

33.    Kiechl S, Willeit J, Poewe W, et al. Insulin sensitivity and regular alcohol consumption: Large, prospective, cross sectional population study (Bruneck study). BMJ 1996;313: 1040-44.

34.    Lazarus R, Sparrow D, Weiss ST. Alcohol intake and insulin levels: The Normative Aging Study. Am J Epidemiol 1997;145:909-16.

35.    Hendriks HF, Veenstra J, Velthuis-te Wierik EJM, Schafsma G, Kluft C. Effect of moderate dose of alcohol with evening meal on fibrinolytic factors. BMJ 1994;308:1003-6.

36.    Pellegrini N, Pareti FI, Stabile F, Brusamolino A, Simonetti P. Effects of moderate

consumption of red wine on platelet aggregation and haemostatic variables in healthy volunteers. Eur J Clin Nutr 1996;50:209-13.

37. Jackson R, Scragg R, Beaglehole R. Does recent alcohol consumption reduce the risk of acute myocardial infarction and coronary death in regular drinkers? Am J Epidemiol 1992; 136:819-24.

38. Dyer AR, Stamler J, Paul O, et al. Alcohol consumption, cardiovascular risk factors, and mortality in two Chicago epidemiologic studies. Circulation 1977;56:1067-74.

39. Wannamethee G, Shaper AG. Alcohol and sudden cardiac death. Br Heart J 1992;68: 443-48.

40. Suhonen O, Aromaa A, Reunanen A, Knekt P. Alcohol consumption and sudden coronary death in middle-aged Finnish men. Acta Med Scand 1987;221:335-41.

41. Poikolainen K. Inebriation and mortality. Int J Epidemiol 1983;12:151-55.

42. Kauhanen J, Kaplan GA, Goldberg DE, Salonen JT. Beer binging and mortality: results from the Kuopio ischaemic heart disease study, a prospective population based study. BMJ 1997;315:846-51.

43. Friedman HS. Cardiovascular effects of ethanol. In: Lieber CD, editor. Medical and nutritional complications of alcoholism: Mechanisms and management. New York: Plenum Medical Book Company, 1992:359-401.

44. Arkwright PD, Beilin LJ, Rouse I, Armstrong BK, Vandongen R. Effects of alcohol use and other aspects of lifestyle on blood pressure levels and prevalence of hypertension in a working population. Circulation 1982;66:60-66.

45. Keil U, Swales JD, Grobbee DE. Alcohol intake and its relation to hypertension. In: Verschuren PM, editor. Health issues related to alcohol consumption. Brussels: ILSI Europe, 1993:17-42.

46. Gruchow HW, Hoffman RG, Aucheson AJ, Barboriak JJ. Effects of drinking patterns on the relationship between alcohol and coronary occlusion, Atherosclerosis 1982;43: 393-404.

47. Koskinen P, Kupari M. Alcohol and cardiac arrhythmias: Patients with unexplained tachyarrhythmias should be questioned about their drinking, BMJ 1992;304:1394-95.

48. DePetrillo PB, White KV, Liu M, Hommer D, Goldman D. Effects of alcohol use and gender on the dynamics of EKG time-series data. Alcohol Clin Exp Res 1999;23: 745-50.

49. Criqui MH. Alcohol and hypertension: New insights from population studies. Eur Heart J 1987;8(Suppl.B):73-85.

50. Kaplan HI, Sadock BJ. Kaplan and Sadock's synopsis of psychiatry. Eighth ed. Baltimore, MD: Williams and Wilkins, 1998.

51. Prescott CA, Kendler KS. Age at first drink and risk of alcoholism: A noncausal association. Alcohol Clin Exp Res 1999;23:101-7.

52. Andréasson S, Allebeck P. Alcohol and psychiatric illness: Longitudinal study of psychiatric admissions in a cohort of Swedish conscripts. Int J Addict 1991;26:713-28.

53. Lazarus NB, Kaplan GA, Cohen RD, Leu D-J. Change in alcohol consumption and risk of death from all causes and from ischaemic heart disease. BMJ 1991;303:553-56.

54. Poikolainen K. Alcohol and mortality: A review. J Clin Epidemiol 1995;48:455-65.

# MODERATE ALCOHOL CONSUMPTION AND RISK OF STROKE: UPDATE ON RECENT EPIDEMIOLOGICAL FINDINGS

Meir J. Stampfer

## Introduction

The epidemiologic evidence regarding the relation between stroke and alcohol consumption has been extensively reviewed by van Gijn et al. [1]; that detailed 1993 review covered studies reported up to 1992. It is instructive to review studies published since that review and to assess whether the weight of evidence or conclusions reached in that previous review have shifted. For total stroke, van Gijn et al. came to the conclusion that there was no association between moderate alcohol consumption and overall risk of total stroke, but an increase at the highest levels of drinking. They noted the possibility of a modest decrease in risk at levels of one to two drinks per day [1]. However, total stroke is heterogeneous, and risk factors for cerebral infarction, caused by an embolus or thrombus, can be quite different from cerebral hemorrhage or subarachnoid hemorrhage. Although some risk factors, notably hypertension and cigarette smoking, are shared among these three stroke types, there is clear evidence that alcohol acts differently. Therefore, studies of total stroke which do not distinguish the types are of limited utility in learning about the specific impact of alcohol. In most western countries, depending on the age distribution, perhaps three quarters or so of total stroke are cerebral infarctions. Thus, data on total stroke in those settings will largely reflect cerebral infarction. The less common cerebral hemorrhage and subarachnoid hemorrhage are more likely to be fatal, so that the distribution of the types among fatal strokes is often different than for nonfatal stroke.

Several major epidemiologic studies examining alcohol and total stroke have been published since the van Gijn review. Most of these support the prior conclusion for a lack of a material association between moderate drinking and risk of total stroke. In their prospective study of Chinese men, Ross et al. [2] and Yuan et al. [3] found no association between moderate drinking and risk of fatal stroke, but do find that more than four drinks per day was associated with an increased risk. In this study, it is likely that a large proportion of the fatal strokes were hemorrhagic. Thun followed one half a million men and women in the U.S. after ascertaining typical alcohol intake. In that study, a modest reduction of total stroke mortality was observed with moderate levels of consumption, and even with higher levels, no increase in risk was observed [4]. One may speculate that the differences in the results from these two studies might be due to the different distribution

89

*R. Paoletti et al. (eds.), Moderate Alcohol Consumption and Cardiovascular Disease,* 89–94.

of stroke types in China and the U.S. This underscores the need to distinguish stroke type in epidemiologic research. Overall, the data continued to support the original conclusion of van Gijn of no increase in risk, and perhaps a modest reduction, associated with moderate alcohol consumption [1].

## Cerebral Infarction

The 1993 review found that any increase in risk of cerebral infarction with moderate alcohol consumption could be confidently excluded but doubt remained as to the evidence suggesting a reduction in risk with moderate consumption [1]. It is in this area that the weight of new evidence forces a reconsideration of that conclusion. In particular, with better assessment of moderate alcohol consumption and distinct categorization of stroke types, most recent studies point clearly toward a reduction in risk of cerebral infarction among moderate alcohol consumers.

In a small hospital based case-control study in Finland, Palomäki et al. found a relative risk of 0.12 (95% CI 0.02-0.65) for light consumption, up to 150 g alcohol per week, with regular consumption. For the next category, 150-300 g per week, the relative risk was 0.55 (95% CI 0.14-2.08). Above that level, which would be greater than four drinks per day, these investigators found an increased risk, particularly among those who binged [5].

In a Swedish study, Hansagi et al. found a significant reduction in risk of cerebral infarction among women with light drinking patterns. For those up to 5 g a day, the relative risk was 0.6 (95% CI 0.5-0.8). No material association was observed among men [6].

Truelsen and colleagues studied weekly alcohol consumption and risk of stroke in the Copenhagen City Heart Study [7]. They found that moderate levels of consumption, from one to 41 drinks per week were associated with a modestly lower risk as compared to those drinking less than once per week. The abstainers (as compared to those drinking 1 to 7 times per week) had an apparent 17% increase in risk. This study followed 13,329 men and women for 16 years, and 752 strokes [7].

The Alpha-Tocopherol Beta-Carotene (ATBC) trial in Finland has also provided useful information regarding alcohol consumption and stroke incidence among male smokers. In this group of 26,556 men followed for an average of 6 years, 733 cases of cerebral infarction were diagnosed. Compared to nondrinkers, light drinkers had only a slight, nonsignificant reduction in risk (RR = 0.91, 95% CI 0.7-1.14). Light drinking was defined as up to two drinks per day. Among heavy drinkers, more than 5 drinks per day, a significant increase in risk was observed [8].

Caicoya and colleagues recently reported results of a community based case-control study of stroke in Spain, including 375 cerebral infarctions. In this setting, a marked reduction in risks was observed for drinkers of up to 30 g per day. In this group, the relative risk was 0.53 (95% CI 0.35-0.80) compared to never-drinkers [9]. As others have observed, there was a trend of increasing risk with high levels of intake. One may speculate that the stronger apparent protection of moderate alcohol consumption in this case-control study as compared to the ATBC cohort might possibly be attributable to a more steady pattern of regular moderate consumption in Spain as compared to a less regular pattern of drinking among the Finnish smokers.

A U.S. case-control study was also reported in 1999 by Sacco et al. [10]. This was a multiethnic population in northern Manhattan, and focused solely on ischemic strokes (n = 677). Cases were matched to community controls derived through random digit dialing. This study also found a similar marked reduction in risk for those with moderate consumption defined as up to two drinks per day. The multivariate adjusted odds ratio was 0.51 (95% CI 0.39-0.67) [10]. Like the two previously discussed studies [8,9], Sacco et al. found an increase in risk among those with heavy alcohol consumption: individuals drinking seven or more drinks per day had nearly triple the risk of ischemic stroke [10].

A fourth major study was also reported in 1999. Berger et al. followed the 22,000 U.S. male physicians participating in the Physicians' Health Study for an average of 12 years or occurrence of stroke. In this analysis, the comparison group constituted those drinking less than once per week. For those with one or more drinks per week, the multivariate adjusted relative risk was 0.77 (95% CI 0.63-0.94) [11]. It is possible that use of the open-ended category of one or more drink per week provides an underestimate of the benefit of regular moderate consumption. Although the overall results were less striking than the previous studies, a statistically significant reduction in risk was observed.

The recent reports on the effect of moderate alcohol consumption on risk of ischemic stroke have added considerable new and reliable data. With a more careful categorization of alcohol consumption, and documentation of cerebral infarction, more consistent findings have emerged than was previously apparent from the early studies. Further supportive information comes from the Bruneck Study, which examined in a cross-sectional sex and age stratified random sample, the relation between alcohol consumption and changes in carotid atherosclerosis. Light drinkers had substantially lower risk than either heavy drinkers or abstainers for progression of carotid atherosclerosis. Compared to moderate drinkers, abstainers had almost two-fold increased risk of incident atherosclerosis in the carotid artery. Likewise, heavier drinkers also had increased risk. Thus, this study using an intermediate marker provides useful corroborating evidence to the cohort and the case-control studies previously described [12]. Taken together with evidence from the earlier literature, one may reasonably now conclude that light to moderate regular drinking is associated with a protective effect on ischemic stroke. Indeed, the evidence is sufficiently large that we should include this benefit in assessing the overall risk and benefits of moderate alcohol consumption.

## Hemorrhagic Stroke

Hemorrhagic stroke includes cerebral hemorrhage and subarachnoid hemorrhage. These are distinct entities with different distributions of incidence and different patterns of risk factors. The previous review of van Gijn et al. [1] concluded that there was little or no relation between moderate alcohol consumption and risk of either of these types of stroke, but higher levels of alcohol were clearly related to increased risks. The recent epidemiological studies of these associations have, in general, tended to confirm those conclusions.

## Subarachnoid Hemorrhage

For subarachnoid hemorrhage, Longstreth et al. reported on 149 cases and 298 matched controls in the state of Washington. Those who drank up to one drink per day had a relative risk of 0.7 (95% CI 0.4-1.1) compared to nondrinkers. Those with one to two drinks per day had a nonsignificant increase in risk, with a relative risk of 1.5 (95% CI 0.7-3.0) [13]. As found in many previous studies, heavier drinkers had significant increase in risk. Adjustment for cigarette smoking tended to attenuate the relative risks.

Juvela et al. studied effects of short-term consumption of alcohol in relation to subarachnoid hemorrhage among 278 cases and 314 controls in Finland. After adjusting for age, hypertension and smoking, recent moderate consumption (up to 40 g within the last 24 hours) was associated with lower risk in both men (RR = 0.3) and women (RR = 0.4). As expected, heavier drinking increased the risk [14]. In the Physicians' Health Study, the relative risk for hemorrhagic stroke was 0.9 (95% CI 0.55-1.54) for those with one or more drinks per week [11]. It is unclear whether this category is a combination of subarachnoid hemorrhage and cerebral hemorrhage. Although the category of drinking was open-ended, most participants were light to moderate drinkers, so this provides further evidence of lack of an adverse effect at low levels of consumption. The ATBC study, cited earlier, also examined subarachnoid hemorrhage, but the number of cases was small. Compared to nondrinkers, light drinkers has no increase in risk, with a relative risk of 1.00 (95% CI 0.47-2.13). There was a gradient with increasing risk beyond the level of light drinking defined as up to two drinks per day [8].

## Intracerebral Hemorrhage

For intracerebral hemorrhage, the most recent findings also tend to support the earlier conclusions of no increase in risk with moderate consumption, but higher risk with higher levels of consumption. For example, in a subsequent study, Juvela et al. studied 156 patients with intracerebral hemorrhage and 332 controls. In examining alcohol intake in the previous 24 hours, as with subarachnoid hemorrhage, the risk intracerebral hemorrhage was lower among moderate drinkers, with a relative risk of 0.33 (95% CI 0.16-0.72). For use in the week before onset of symptoms, apart from the preceding 24 hours, the adjusted relative risk was 2.0 (95% CI 1.0-3.5) for up to 150 g [15]. In Sweden, Hansagi et al. examined 195 cases of hemorrhagic stroke and found no relation with intake of alcohol [6]. This was a moderate drinking cohort and the study had inadequate power to detect risks associated with heavy drinking. Nonetheless, it adds important evidence providing further reassurance as to the lack of an increased risk at moderate levels of consumption. Similar findings were observed in the ATBC for intracerebral hemorrhage compared to nondrinkers, light drinkers had a relative risk of 0.83 (95% CI 0.45-1.50), with an increase in risk observed among heavy drinkers [8]. In the Spanish case-control study cited earlier [9] a similar pattern emerged with nonsignificant reductions in risk with low to moderate levels of consumption. For example, for those drinking less than 30 g per day, the relative risk was 0.88 (95% CI 0.44-1.74). They also observed, as did most other studies, that heavy drinking increased the risk. In this study, alcohol intake greater than 140 g per day was associated with more than a six-fold increase in risk [9]. In Australia, Thrift et al. also observed a nonsignificant reduction in risk of intracerebral hemorrhage with moderate alcohol consumption with a relative risk of 0.7 (95% CI 0.4-1.2) [16]. This was in contrast to a three-fold increase in risk with heavy drinking in this study of 331 case-control pairs.

Results from studies of intracerebral hemorrhage are remarkably consistent. In virtually every instance, investigators have observed either a modest nonsignificant decrease in risk, or no association for moderate levels of consumption. Consistent findings demonstrate an elevated risk for heavy drinkers.

## Conclusions

Review of the recent epidemiologic findings regarding alcohol and stroke has largely confirmed previous conclusions, particularly regarding subarachnoid hemorrhage and intracerebral hemorrhage. The most recent data strongly confirm previous conclusions of lack of an increased risk of either type of stroke with moderate alcohol consumption, but a clear increase in risk with heavy use. In contrast, the recent epidemiologic data has provided a sound basis for altering previous conclusions regarding ischemic stroke. Although the suspicion of a potential reduction in risk had been raised for many years, the prior evidence had not been persuasive. More recent epidemiologic studies have consistently observed a reduction in risk with moderate levels of consumption, and in view of the shared risk factors with coronary disease, where a benefit for moderate alcohol has been established, we may now regard the apparent benefit for ischemic stroke in a similar light, though less well substantiated. Thus, in evaluating risks and benefits of moderate alcohol consumption, one should include the substantial reduction in risk of ischemic stroke among the benefits, and one can, with confidence, exclude concerns about an increase in risk of intracerebral hemorrhage or subarachnoid hemorrhage, so long as the intake is strictly kept within the bounds of moderation.

## References

1.      van Gijn J, Stampfer MJ, Wolfe C, Algra A. The association between alcohol and stroke. In: Verschuren PM, editor. Health issues related to alcohol consumption. Washington: ILSI Press, 1993: 43-79.

2.      Ross RK, Yuan JM, Henderson BE, Park J, Gao YT, Yu MC. Prospective evaluation of the dietary and other predictors of fatal stroke in Shanghai, China. Circulation 1997;96(1): 50-55.

3.      Yuan J, Ross R, Gao Y, Henderson B, Yu M. Follow up study of moderate alcohol intake

and mortality among middle aged men in Shanghai, China. BMJ 1997;314:18-23.

4.    Thun M, Peto R, Lopez A, Monaco J, Henley S, Heath CJ, et al. Alcohol consumption and mortality among middle-aged and elderly U.S. adults. N Engl J Med 1997;337(24):1705-14.

5.    Palomaki H, Kaste M. Regular light-to-moderate intake of alcohol and the risk of ischemic stroke. Is there a beneficial effect? Stroke 1993;24:1828-32.

6.    Hansagi H, Romelsjo A, Gerhardsson de Verdier M, Andreasson S, Leifman A. Alcohol consumption and stroke mortality. 20-year follow-up of 15,077 men and women. Stroke 1995;26:1768-73.

7.    Truelsen T, Gronbaek M, Schnohr P, Boysen G. Intake of beer, wine and spirits and risk of stroke: The Copenhagen City Heart Study. Stroke 1998;29:2467-72.

8.    Leppala J, Paunio M, Virtamo J, Fogelholm R, Albanes D, Taylor P, et al. Alcohol consumption and stroke incidence in male smokers. Circulation 1999;100:1209-14.

9.    Caicoya M, Rodriguez T, Corrales C, Cuello R, Lasheras C. Alcohol and stroke: A community case-control study in Asturias, Spain. J Clin Epidemiol 1999;52(7):677-84.

10.   Sacco R, Elkind M, Boden-Albala B, IF L, Kargman D, Hauser W, et al. The protective effect of moderate alcohol consumption on ischemic stroke. JAMA 1999;281:53-60.

11.   Berger K, Ajani U, Kase C, Gaziano M, Buring J, Glynn R, et al. Light-to-moderate alcohol consumption and the risk of stroke among US male physicians. N Engl J Med 1999;341:1557-64.

12.   Kiechl S, Willeit J, Rungger G, Egger G, Oberhollenzer F, Bonora E. Alcohol consumption and atherosclerosis: What is the relation? Stroke 1998;29:900-907.

13.   Longstreth WT, Jr., Nelson LM, Koepsell TD, van Belle G. Cigarette smoking, alcohol use, and subarachnoid hemorrhage. Stroke 1992;23:1242-49.

14.   Juvela S, Hillbom M, Numminen H, Koskinen P. Cigarette smoking and alcohol consumption as risk factors for aneurysmal subarachnoid hemorrhage. Stroke 1993;24:639-46.

15.   Juvela S, Hillbom M, Palomaki H. Risk factors for spontaneous intracerebral hemorrhage. Stroke 1995;26:1558-64.

16.   Thrift A, Donnan G, McNeil J. Heavy drinking, but not moderate or intermediate drinking, increases the risk of intracerebral hemorrhage. Epidemiology 1999;10(3):307-12.

# WHAT INFLUENCES THE RELATIONSHIP BETWEEN ALCOHOL CONSUMPTION AND TOTAL MORTALITY?

Michael J. Thun, Jane Henley, and Aron Rosenthal

## Introduction

Alcohol consumption can increase death rates from injuries, violence, suicide, poisoning, cirrhosis of the liver, certain cancers, and hemorrhagic stroke, but can decrease death rates from coronary heart disease and thrombotic stroke. The net balance of risks and benefits varies according to the amount and pattern of drinking, and may differ across age, gender, and other characteristics of the population. This presentation examines factors that influence the net relationship of alcohol consumption to all-cause mortality rates.

## Methods

In the large American Cancer Society cohort, Cancer Prevention Study II (CPS-II) [1], we first identified factors that modify the relationship between drinking and all-cause mortality at various levels of alcohol consumption. These included the amount and pattern of drinking and various characteristics of drinkers that modify the background prevalence of conditions affected by alcohol. The size of CPS-II (nearly 490,000 adults and over 46,000 deaths in the analytic cohort) provides fairly precise risk estimates within narrow ranges of self-reported alcohol consumption. CPS-II also illustrates some of the limitations of exposure classification and generalizability shared by nearly all cohort studies of alcohol consumption and mortality.

Next we conducted an overview of all published epidemiologic studies that provided data on annual all-cause mortality rates among men or women who report "moderate" average alcohol consumption. We defined "moderate" drinking as average consumption of one drink daily in women or 1-2 drinks per day in men [2]. Most studies gave only the relative risk of death from all causes at this level of drinking compared to the death rate in nondrinkers. We estimated 95% confidence intervals (CI) based on inverse variance for the total number of deaths. We hypothesized that three factors might contribute to heterogeneity across these studies: the contribution of cardiovascular diseases as a percentage of all deaths; the prevalence of "binge" drinking in adults; and the percentage of total alcohol consumed as spirits. From most of the studies we could calculate coronary heart disease (CHD) as a percentage of all deaths. We used country- and calendar year-

95

*R. Paoletti et al. (eds.), Moderate Alcohol Consumption and Cardiovascular Disease, 95–103.*
© 2000 *Kluwer Academic Publishers and Fondazione Giovanni Lorenzini. Printed in the Netherlands.*

specific historical data on sales of alcoholic beverages as an ecological index of spirit consumption [3].

## Results

In CPS-II, a curvilinear relationship is evident between the average quantity of alcohol consumed and all-cause death rates during the nine-year follow-up (Figure 1) [1]. Men and women who, at baseline, reported an average of one drink daily experienced approximately 20% lower annual death rates than did abstainers. This survival advantage associated with moderate drinking diminished with heavier drinking. The death rates shown in Figure 1 represent average death rates among the predominantly middle-aged and elderly, educated, middle-class study population. The rates are adjusted for age, tobacco smoking, diet, and other factors. However, the pattern associating alcohol consumption with all-cause mortality differs in different populations, as discussed below.

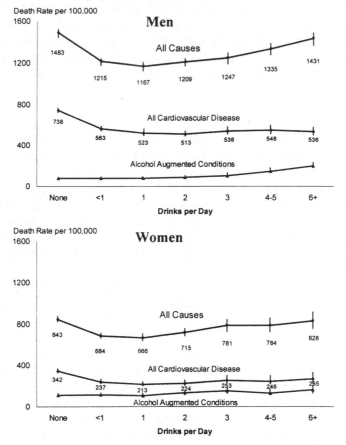

Figure 1. CPS-II death rates by drink per day.

CPS-II also illustrates several general principles regarding the relationship between alcohol consumption and all-cause mortality. First, the potential impact of drinking on specific conditions, and thereby on all-cause death rates, is shown better by absolute rates than by relative risk. For example, CPS-II men who drink an average of four or more alcoholic drinks daily experience death rates from cirrhosis or alcoholism more than seven times (RR = 7.5, 95% CI = 4.9-11.4) higher than the rate of nondrinkers. The same level of drinking is associated with a 30% percent reduction in cardiovascular death rates (RR = 0.7, 95% CI = 0.7-0.8). In absolute terms, however, cardiovascular conditions account for ten times as many deaths (n = 1563) as cirrhosis and alcoholism (151) among the CPS-II men who reported four or more drinks daily in 1982. The 30% reduction in cardiovascular death rates associated with "moderate" drinking thus has a larger absolute impact on all cause death rates than does the increase in cirrhosis and alcoholism, even at this level of drinking.

A second principle illustrated in CPS-II is that the greater the contribution of cardiovascular conditions to all cause mortality, the greater the reduction in both absolute and relative risk associated with moderate drinking. This pattern is more easily seen for relative than for absolute risk. In Figure 2, the all-cause RR estimates associated with each level of drinking are lower for participants age 60-79 than for those age 30-59. The same is true for persons at high, compared to low, background risk of cardiovascular death, due to previous cardiovascular morbidity or risk factors (discussed below). The potential benefit of moderate regular alcohol consumption for cardiovascular risk has the greatest impact on all cause death rates in populations where cardiovascular disease contributes a large fraction of all deaths. Age is one characteristic that dramatically increases the background risk of cardiovascular disease. Among males age 15 to 29 in the U.S., cardiovascular conditions comprise only 4% of all deaths, compared to 46% of all deaths in men age 60 and above, based on 1990 rates [4]. The opposite is seen for deaths from injury, violence, suicide, and other external causes, which contribute 75% of all deaths among U.S. males age 15 to 29 in 1990, but only 3% among men age 60 and above. The age-related increase in cardiovascular mortality (thought to benefit from moderate alcohol consumption), together with the age-related decrease in deaths from external causes (affected adversely by alcohol consumption) work together to shift the balance of potential risks and benefits with aging.

Figure 2 also suggests that preexisting cardiovascular disease (history of a heart attack, stroke, hypertension, diabetes, or medications for these) may qualitatively change the shape of the dose-response relationship between alcohol consumption and all-cause mortality. A J-shaped relationship is seen with increasing alcohol consumption among "low risk" men and women age 30-59 (those not reporting cardiovascular morbidity or risk factors at baseline). This changes to a U-shaped relationship in the two subgroups with intermediate background cardiovascular risk, and to an L-shaped relationship among persons age 60-79 at very high cardiovascular risk.

CPS-II illustrates several limitations shared by most of the epidemiologic studies of alcohol consumption and mortality. These involve misclassification of exposure, the potential for residual confounding by factors associated with alcohol consumption, and issues of generalizability. People who report drinking one drink daily, on average, may actually consume seven drinks each Saturday. Those who report no alcohol consumption presently or for the past ten years may have been heavy drinkers prior to that. As in any observational (nonrandomized) study, associations with alcohol consumption may reflect incompletely controlled confounding by factors that are associated with alcohol consumption. Constraints on generalizability of the CPS-II findings are that the population only includes adults, age 30 and above. It excludes or underrepresents certain high-risk groups such as adolescents, young adults, binge drinkers, or very heavy drinkers, very poor people, or groups in which deaths from external causes outnumber deaths from cardiovascular disease.

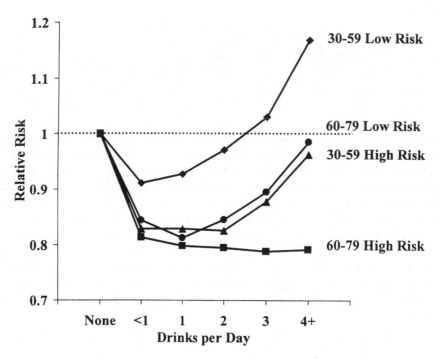

Figure 2. Relative risk of all-cause mortality by alcohol consumption, age, and cardiovascular risk, CPS-II men and women combined.

**Overview of Published Epidemiologic Studies**

We identified 31 published studies that provided data on "moderate" alcohol consumption and all-cause mortality. Sixteen of these were from the United States [1,5-19] five from Great Britain [20-23], one from Australia [24], three from Scandinavia [25-27], and seven from other countries in Western Europe [28-30], Eastern Europe [31], the former Soviet Union [19], China [32], and Japan [33]. One study [19] provided data on both the United States and Russia. We excluded six studies from our analysis: two in which the cohort overlapped with another study [12,34], two that presented only combined data for men and women [14,15], and two that did not meet our criteria for moderate drinking [26,30].

Figure 3 plots the relative risk for all-cause mortality associated with moderate drinking in 24 published studies of men. In general, the relative risk of death from all causes during the follow-up in these studies is below 1.0 in "moderate" drinkers and decreases the greater the contribution of CHD to all deaths. Four studies found atypical increases in overall death rates associated with "moderate" drinking. The three shown in Figure 3 were conducted in Finland, Russia, and the former Yugoslavia, where binge drinking among adults is reputedly common. A fourth study by Andreasson found an even larger increase in all cause death rates among military recruits in Sweden [25]. This is not included in Figure 3, because data were not provided on CHD as a percentage of all deaths. Like the other studies from Scandinavia and Eastern Europe, it may misclassify binge drinking by expressing consumption only as an average. Two studies reported atypically low RR estimates with "moderate" drinking: that by Yuan et al. in China [32] and by Keil et al. in Germany [29]. We have no explanation other than chance for why these studies may be atypical. A similar trend in the all cause RR with much less scatter is seen when only the sixteen U.S. studies are graphed separately (figure not shown).

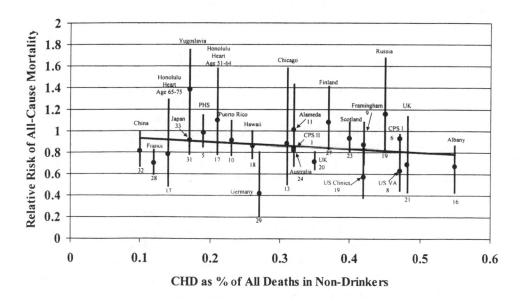

Figure 3. All-cause RR from "moderate" drinking by CHD as percent of all deaths for men—world.

Figure 4 shows the graph of all-cause relative risk associated with "moderate" alcohol consumption in women. Unexpectedly, the slope of this relationship increases rather than decreases with the percentage of all deaths contributed by CHD. This increase is due entirely to three studies from Russia [19], Australia [24], and Alameda County, California [11]. Although it is not clear why the slope of the relationship in women goes in the opposite direction from that predicted, one possibility is that because alcohol consumption is less socially acceptable among women than men in many cultures, solitary or sporadic drinking among women may be misclassified as regular moderate drinking.

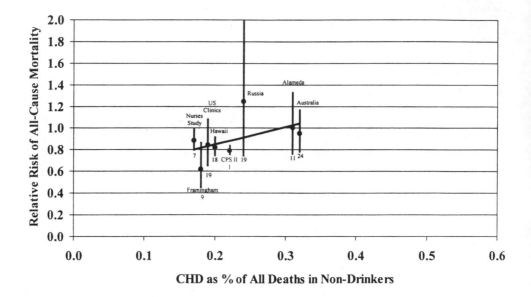

Figure 4. All-cause RR from "moderate" drinking by CHD as percent of all deaths for women—world.

## Discussion

Our analyses identify several factors that modify the net relationship between alcohol consumption and all cause death rates. As expected, the amount of alcohol consumed and the pattern of drinking (binge or regular) are highly correlated with death rates from conditions that are exacerbated by alcohol consumption, particularly injuries, violence, certain alcohol-related cancers, and liver cirrhosis. The detrimental effects of binge and extremely heavy drinking are not well studied in most of the existing cohort studies, yet these are likely to contribute to some of the heterogeneity across studies. In contrast, the type of alcohol consumed (at least ecological data reflecting the percentage of alcohol consumed as spirits) did not appear to modify the association between alcohol and all-cause death rates in our analyses of these studies.

Two characteristics of drinkers, age and male sex, affect the background risk of both cardiovascular diseases and of death from external causes (motor vehicle accidents, violence, etc.). In general, the larger the fraction of all deaths contributed by cardiovascular conditions, and the smaller the percentage contributed by external causes, the larger the potential benefit of "moderate" drinking on all-cause mortality. The presence of preexisting cardiovascular disease may have the additional effect of modifying the dose-response relationship between alcohol consumption and cardiovascular as well as all-cause mortality.

## Issues for Future Research

The following questions could be addressed in future research:

- Why does the relationship between "moderate" average alcohol consumption and all-cause mortality appear different in women than men in several studies [24,19,11]?
- Are drinking patterns misclassified more often in women than in men (perhaps because of social taboos, more solitary drinking, smaller body size)?
- What is the net impact of "moderate" alcohol consumption in women at high risk of breast cancer but low risk of cardiovascular disease?
- To what extent does "moderate" drinking affect accidental injuries or deaths?
- To what extent does "moderate" drinking affect the risk of aerodigestive tract cancers in smokers?
- What are the effects of "moderate" drinking in diabetes?
- Could the cardioprotective effect of alcohol be mimicked by a drug that did not cause intoxication or breast cancer?
- What is the net impact of moderate drinking in women who are at high risk of breast cancer and low risk of vascular disease?

## References

1.      Thun MJ, Peto R, Lopez AD, et al. Alcohol consumption and mortality among middle-aged and elderly U.S. adults [see comments]. N Engl J Med 1997;337:1705-14.
2.      Nutrition and Your Health: Dietary Guidelines for Americans. Washington D.C.: U.S. Department of Agriculture U.S. Department of Health and Human Resources, 1995.
3.      World Drink Trends. Henley-on-Thames: NTC Publications Ltd., 1998.
4.      Table 1-27: Deaths from 282 selected causes, by 5-year age groups, race, and sex: United States, 1990. National Center for Health Statistics. Vital Statistics of the United States, 1990. Vol. 2 Mortality. Part A. Washington, D.C.: Government Printing Office, 1994:312-71. (DHHS publication no. (PHS) 95-1101.).
5.      Camargo CA, Hennekens CH, Gaziano JM, Glynn RJ, Manson JE, Stampfer MJ. Prospective study of moderate alcohol consumption and mortality in U.S. male physicians.

Arch Int Med 1997;157:79-85.

6.    Boffetta P, Garfinkel L. Alcohol drinking and mortality among men enrolled in an American Cancer Society prospective study [see comments]. Epidemiology 1990;1:342-48.

7.    Fuchs CS, Stampfer MJ, Colditz GA, et al. Alcohol consumption and mortality among women [see comments] [published erratum appears in N Engl J Med 1997 Feb 13;336(7): 523]. N Engl J Med 1995;332:1245-50.

8.    de Labry LO, Glynn RJ, Levenson MR, Hermos JA, LoCastro JS, Vokonas PS. Alcohol consumption and mortality in an American male population: recovering the U-shaped curve—findings from the normative Aging Study. J Studies on Alcohol. 1992;53:25-32.

9.    Friedman LA, Kimball AW. Coronary heart disease mortality and alcohol consumption in Framingham. Am J Epidemiol 1986;124:481-89.

10.   Kittner SJ, Garcia-Palmieri MR, Costas R, Jr, Cruz-Vidal M, Abbott RD, Havlik RJ. Alcohol and coronary heart disease in Puerto Rico. Am J Epidemiol 1983;117:538-50.

11.   Lazarus NB, Kaplan GA, Cohen RD, Leu DJ. Change in alcohol consumption and risk of death from all causes and from ischaemic heart disease. Br Med J 1991;303:553-56.

12.   Camacho TC, Kaplan GA, Cohen RD. Alcohol consumption and mortality in Alameda County. J Chronic Dis 1987;40:229-36.

13.   Dyer AR, Stamler J, Paul O, et al. Alcohol consumption and 17-year mortality in the Chicago Western Electric Company study. Preven Med 1980;9:78-90.

14.   Colditz GA, Branch LG, Lipnick RJ, et al. Moderate alcohol and decreased cardiovascular mortality in an elderly cohort. Am Heart J 1985;109:886-89.

15.   Klatsky AL, Friedman GD, Siegelaub AB. Alcohol and mortality. A ten-year Kaiser-Permanente experience. Ann Int Med 1981;95:139-45.

16.   Gordon T, Doyle JT. Drinking and mortality. The Albany Study. Am J Epidemiol 1987; 125:263-70.

17.   Goldberg RJ, Burchfiel CM, Reed DM, Wergowske G, Chiu D. A prospective study of the health effects of alcohol consumption in middle-aged and elderly men. The Honolulu Heart Program. Circulation 1994;89:651-59.

18.   Maskarinec G, Meng L, Kolonel LN. Alcohol intake, body weight, and mortality in a multiethnic prospective cohort. Epidemiology 1998;9:654-61.

19.   Deev A, Shestov D, Abernathy J, Kapustina A, Muhina N, Irving S. Association of alcohol consumption to morality in middle-aged U.S. and Russian men and women. Ann Epidemiol 1998;8:147-53.

20.   Doll R, Peto R, Hall E, Wheatley K, Gray R. Mortality in relation to consumption of alcohol: 13 years' observations on male British doctors [see comments]. Br Med J 1994; 309:911-18.

21.   Marmot MG, Rose G, Shipley M J, Thomas BJ. Alcohol and mortality: A U-shaped curve. Lancet 1981;1:580-83.

22.   Wannamethee SG, Shaper AG. Lifelong teetotalers, ex-drinkers and drinkers: Mortality and the incidence of major coronary heart disease events in middle-aged British men. Int J Epidemiol 1997;26:523-31.

23.   Hart CL, Smith GD, Hole DJ, Hawthorne VM. Alcohol consumption and mortality from all causes, coronary heart disease, and stroke: Results from a prospective cohort study of Scottish men with 21 years of follow up. Br Med J 1999;318:1725-29.

24.   Cullen KJ, Knuiman MW, Ward NJ. Alcohol consumption and mortality in Busselton, Western Australia. Am J Epidemiol 1993;137:242-48.

25. Andreasson S Allebeck P Romelsjo A. Alcohol and mortality among young men: longitudinal study of Swedish conscripts. Br Med J Clin Res Ed 1988;296:1021-25.

26. Salonen JT, Puska P, Nissinen A. Intake of spirits and beer and risk of myocardial infarction and death--a longitudinal study in Eastern Finland. J Chronic Dis 1983;36:533-43.

27. Suhonen O, Aromaa A, Reunanen A, Knekt P. Alcohol consumption and sudden coronary death in middle-aged Finnish men. Acta Med Scand 1987;221:335-41.

28. Renaud SC, Gueguen R, Schenker J, d'Houtaud A. Alcohol and mortality in middle-aged men from eastern France. Epidemiology 1998;9:184-88.

29. Keil U, Chambless LE, Doring A, Filipiak B, Stieber J. The relation of alcohol intake to coronary heart disease and all-cause mortality in a beer-drinking population [see comments]. Epidemiology 1997;8:150-56.

30. Farchi G, Fidanza F, Mariotti S, Menotti A. Alcohol and mortality in the Italian rural cohorts of the Seven Countries Study. Int J Epidemiol 1992;21:74-81.

31. Kozararevic D, McGee D, Vojvodic N, et al. Frequency of alcohol consumption and morbidity and mortality: The Yugoslavia Cardiovascular Disease Study. Lancet 1980;1:613-16.

32. Yuan JM, Ross RK, Gao YT, Henderson BE, Yu MC. Follow up study of moderate alcohol intake and mortality among middle aged men in Shanghai, China [see comments]. Br Med J 1997;314:18-23.

33. Kono S, Ikeda M, Tokudome S, Nishizumi M, Kuratsune M. Alcohol and mortality: A cohort study of male Japanese physicians. Int J Epidemiol 1986;15:527-32.

34. Shaper AG, Wannamethee G, Walker M. Alcohol and mortality in British men: Explaining the U-shaped curve [see comments]. Lancet 1988;2:1267-73.

# EPIDEMIOLOGICAL CONFOUNDERS IN THE RELATIONSHIP BETWEEN ALCOHOL AND CARDIOVASCULAR DISEASE

A. Gerald Shaper and S. Goya Wannamethee

## Introduction

In almost all epidemiological studies of alcohol and cardiovascular disease, non-drinking status is associated with increased risk compared with light or moderate alcohol intake, resulting in a J- or U-shaped curve relating alcohol intake to disease outcome. In populations with low average alcohol intake the relationship may be inverse. The usual interpretation is that the lowest point on such curves (light or moderate drinking) represents optimum exposure to alcohol and that the increased risk in non-drinkers reflects the consequence of suboptimal exposure, i.e. not consuming sufficient alcohol to produce benefit. J- or U-shaped curves for mortality are also seen with serum total cholesterol and body mass index and in both of these examples the increased mortality in the lower extreme of the distribution has been shown to be due in the main, to confounding by pre-existing ill health and disadvantageous risk factors [1,2 ].

We have previously shown that changes take place in alcohol drinking behavior with increasing age, and that there is a drift from heavy and moderate drinking towards non-drinking affected to a considerable extent by ill health and medication [3,4 ]. Reducing or giving up alcohol is associated with higher rates of new diagnoses and higher rates of cardiovascular and non-cardiovascular mortality than remaining stable [5]. As a consequence, non-drinkers have characteristics likely to increase morbidity and mortality compared with occasional or light drinkers. Also, regular light drinkers have characteristics extremely advantageous to health [6]. These characteristics produce distorted estimates of the effects of alcohol on cardiovascular disease and all cause mortality.

In this paper, we present new data on the changes taking place in alcohol intake over time and on the effects that classification of intake at different time periods (i.e. different ages) have on the alcohol-mortality relationship. We also examine the characteristics of those who remain stable and those who change their intake over time and reflect on the extent to which these characteristics account for the observed intake-mortality relationships, i.e. the shape of the curves.

R. Paoletti et al. (eds.), Moderate Alcohol Consumption and Cardiovascular Disease, 105–112.
© 2000 Kluwer Academic Publishers and Fondazione Giovanni Lorenzini. Printed in the Netherlands.

## Subjects and Methods

The material presented in this paper comes from a prospective study of cardiovascular disease in 7,735 men aged 40-59 years at entry recruited from the age-sex registers of one group general practice in each of 24 British towns and examined in 1978-80 (The British Regional Heart Study). The overall response rate was 78% and men with pre-existing cardiovascular disease or on regular medical treatment were not excluded. Research nurses administered to each man a standard questionnaire (Q1) which included questions on smoking, alcohol intake, and medical history. Five years after this initial examination (1983-85) a postal questionnaire (Q5) was sent to all surviving men and detailed information on medical history, changes in smoking and drinking behavior and in other risk factors was obtained from 98% of the survivors. In 1992 and again in 1996, further postal questionnaires were sent to survivors and were completed by 91% and 88% respectively.

### ALCOHOL INTAKE

The men were classified as non-drinkers, occasional drinkers, light (1-15 units/week), moderate (16-42), and heavy (> 42 units/week) drinkers. A U.K. unit is 8-10 grams alcohol. Only from Q5 onwards was it possible to separate lifelong teetotallers (LLTTs) and ex-drinkers (those who had previously been regular drinkers; light, moderate, or heavy). Occasional drinkers are used as the baseline group as we have shown repeatedly that the non-drinking group is an inappropriate standard [3-5].

### LIFE STYLE FACTORS

Social class, smoking, body mass index, and physical activity are based on data from Q1 and/or Q5. Pre-existing disease status is based on recall of doctor diagnoses and regular medication at Q1 and Q5.

### FOLLOW-UP

All men were followed up for all-cause mortality and for cardiovascular morbidity from the initial screening (Q1) and all deaths have been recorded to December 1997 (18.8 years from screening). Follow-up has been achieved in 99% of the cohort

## Results

### CHANGES IN ALCOHOL INTAKE PATTERNS

Over time, there is a decrease in the percentage of men who are moderate or heavy drinkers, an increase in the percentage of non-drinkers and an increase in the proportion of non-drinkers who are ex-drinkers, reaching 74% at 12-14 years after screening (Table 1). The stability of drinking pattern is initially low in moderate and heavy drinkers but it increases with time, i.e. there is a "hard core" of persistent heavier drinkers. Stability is greatest at the lower levels of intake, particularly in non-drinkers.

EFFECT OF INTAKE PATTERNS ON MORTALITY AT DIFFERENT TIME PERIODS

Before examining the patterns of mortality in the alcohol intake groups at different time periods, we need to determine the characteristics of men at these time periods, particularly non-drinkers and light drinkers, so that appropriate adjustments can be made to avoid or diminish confounding (Table 2). All rates are higher in Q92 than Q1 but both at Q1 and Q92, light drinkers have far more favorable characteristics and health patterns than non-drinkers. The difference in cigarette smoking is most marked at Q92.

Table 1. Alcohol intake (%) at screening (Q1), five years later (Q5) and 12-14 years after screening (Q92).

|  | Q1 | Q5 | Q92 |
|---|---|---|---|
| Age range (yrs) | 40-59 | 45-64 | 52-71 |
| Mean age (yrs) | 50 | 55 | 63 |
| TT |  | 4.6 | 4.3 |
| (all non-drinkers) | (6.0) | (9.6) | (16.6) |
| Ex- |  | 5.0 | 12.3 |
| Occasional | 23.9 | 29.4 | 22.9 |
| Light | 32.9 | 36.8 | 39.0 |
| Moderate | 26.4 | 19.1 | 13.8 |
| Heavy | 10.8 | 4.1 | 3.4 |
| Ex/Non (%) | - | (52) | (74) |

Figure 1 shows the relative risks for cardiovascular and total mortality, adjusting first for age only and then for both life style characteristics and pre-existing ill health and regular medication. In the younger middle-aged men (Q1), there is a shallow U-shaped curve for both total and CV mortality. With occasional drinkers as baseline, after full adjustment, there is a significant benefit for cardiovascular disease in moderate drinkers (20-60 gm/day) but not in light drinkers and no benefit for total mortality. In older men, with occasional drinkers as baseline, after full adjustment there is no significant benefit for cardiovascular mortality despite the marked inverse relationship. For total mortality there is a striking U-shaped curve with significantly increased risk in non-drinkers and heavy drinkers. However, if non-drinkers are used as baseline rather than occasional drinkers, there is a considerable apparent benefit for light drinkers seen for both cardiovascular mortality (RR = 0.47; CI 0.34-0.64) and for total mortality (RR = 0.54; CI 0.40-0.74).

Table 2. Characteristics and recall of doctor diagnoses and regular medication (%) in non-drinkers and light drinkers at screening (Q1) and 12-14 years later (Q92).

|  | Q1 | | Q92 | |
|---|---|---|---|---|
|  | Non | Light | Non | Light |
| Age (yrs) | 51.4 | 50.4 | 64.2 | 62.9 |
| Obese | 20.0 | 16.8 | 25.1 | 23.6 |
| Smokers | 36.9 | 33.1 | 23.2 | 13.9 |
| "Active" | 31.5 | 43.8 | 31.2 | 47.3 |
| Manual | 67.5 | 46.7 | 67.3 | 46.7 |
| CHD | 11.2 | 5.1 | 21.6 | 14.5 |
| High BP | 14.6 | 12.3 | 28.0 | 24.8 |
| Stoke | 1.5 | 0.6 | 6.4 | 3.0 |
| Diabetes | 4.1 | 1.8 | 6.3 | 3.8 |
| Medication | 40.8 | 26.3 | 58.1 | 47.2 |

STABLE AND CHANGED DRINKING GROUPS

To what extent are these patterns of alcohol-mortality relationships determined by alterations in alcohol intake over time? To approach this question we have reclassified alcohol intake on the basis of stability and change in intake over the five years between Q1 and Q5:

- Stable (56%): Non-drinkers, occasional, light, and moderate/heavy.
- Changed (44%): Increased to moderate/heavy, became light, became occasional, gave up.
- The increased group were those moving from occasional or light to moderate or heavy. Those who became light drinkers came from occasional and moderate drinkers. Those who became occasional were predominantly light drinkers. Those who gave up drinking were mainly moderate or heavy

drinkers previously.

Using stable occasional as the baseline, Table 3 shows the relative risks of CVD and total mortality over 12 years follow-up from Q5 for the alcohol categories with adjustments first for age (A) and then (B) for age, life style characteristics, and pre-existing disease and medication. Light stable drinkers had the lowest age-adjusted risks of cardiovascular and total mortality. Those who became light drinkers had higher risk than stable light drinkers. Men who had given up drinking between Q1 and Q5 (recent ex-drinkers) had the highest risk of all.

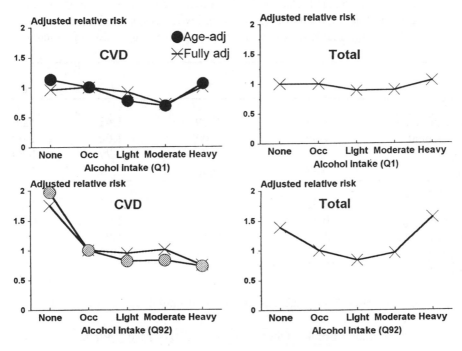

Figure 1. Alcohol intake at screening (Q1) and 12 years later (Q92) and relative risks of cardiovascular and total mortality. O = age-adjusted; X = adjusted for age, smoking social class, BMI, physical activity, and pre-existing disease and medication.

However, stable light drinkers had a far better overall profile than any other group (Table 4) including stable occasional drinkers and those who became light drinkers.. Those who gave up drinking had by far the worst risk factor profile and recent ex-drinkers have a worse profile than long term non-drinkers. Adjustment for these differences in characteristics and health status (Table 3; column B) reduced the benefit for CVD and total mortality in light stable drinkers although they still showed significantly lower risk CVD mortality (but not total mortality) than stable occasional drinkers. Adjustment considerably reduced the CVD and total mortality risk in those who had given up drinking, both recent and long term. The increased risk in those who gave up drinking is almost entirely due to pre-existing disease and medication. Those who became light drinkers showed lower risk of CVD mortality than stable occasional after full adjustment but still showed slightly higher risk than the stable light drinkers. When changes in alcohol intake are not taken into account, the benefit for CVD mortality in light drinkers is much reduced (RR = 0.84;95% CI 0.70-1.20 rather than the RR = 0.69 95% CI 0,54-0.89; see Table 3), presumably because of the combining of stable light drinkers and those who become light drinkers.

Table 3. Stable and changed alcohol intake groups and adjusted relative risks for cardiovascular and total mortality on 12 years follow-up. Adjusted for (A) age, (B) age, smoking, social class, initial BMI, physical activity, pre-existing disease/medication.

|  | Cardiovascular | | Total | |
| --- | --- | --- | --- | --- |
|  | A | B | A | B |
| **Stable** | | | | |
| Non-drinkers | 1.13 | 0.89 | 1.41 | 1.20 |
| Occasional | 1.00 | 1.00 | 1.00 | 1.00 |
| Light | 0.58 * | 0.69 * | 0.77 | 0.89 |
| Mod/heavy | 0.88 | 0.82 | 1.19 | 1.07 |
| **Changed** | | | | |
| Inc to M/H | 0.92 | 1.06 | 0.92 | 1.00 |
| Become Light | 0.86 | 0.79 * | 1.05 | 0.99 |
| Become Occ | 0.84 | 0.77 * | 1.06 | 0.97 |
| Give up | 1.62 | 1.14 | 1.63 | 1.19 |

* p<0.05

Table 4. Characteristics (%) of stable and changed alcohol intake groups (Q5).

|  | Man | Smok | Obese | Active | CHD | Med | P/F health | New CVD |
| --- | --- | --- | --- | --- | --- | --- | --- | --- |
| **Stable** | | | | | | | | |
| Non-drinkers | 67 | 30 | 20 | 33 | 15 | 41 | 32 | 15 |
| Occ | 54 | 30 | 19 | 35 | 9 | 31 | 21 | 10 |
| Light | 41 | 22 | 17 | 47 | 7 | 25 | 15 | 9 |
| Mod/heavy | 62 | 42 | 26 | 35 | 7 | 32 | 26 | 13 |
| **Changed** | | | | | | | | |
| Inc to M/H | 46 | 27 | 27 | 43 | 9 | 26 | 16 | 12 |
| Become L | 64 | 33 | 24 | 38 | 11 | 32 | 24 | 13 |
| Become Occ | 57 | 33 | 23 | 37 | 10 | 34 | 24 | 13 |
| Give up | 72 | 40 | 26 | 27 | 14 | 48 | 44 | 16 |

Man=manual; P/F=poor/fair. New CVD= diagnosis in preceding 5 years

LIFE LONG TEETOTALLERS AND EX-DRINKERS

Thus far, we have combined lifelong teetotallers (LLTT) and ex-drinkers as non-drinkers, as our major concern has been to consider the effects of confounding and the use of occasional drinkers as baseline on the alcohol-mortality relationships. Now, briefly, we will separate non-drinkers into LLTTs and ex-drinkers and examine the relative risk of mortality based on alcohol intakes at Q5 (average age 55 yrs), when half of non-drinkers are ex-drinkers, and Q92 (average age 63 yrs), when three-quarters of non-drinkers are ex-drinkers. Follow-up from Q5 (mean 11.8 years) shows a striking difference between LLTTs and ex-drinkers in both cardiovascular and total mortality, with ex-drinkers having significantly higher risk. Follow-up from Q92 (5 years) shows that both LLTTs and ex-drinkers have a similar high risk of both cardiovascular and total mortality. Whatever the reasons for this observation, and despite the fact that LLTTs tend to have low levels of most established cardiovascular risk factors, these findings emphasizes the unsuitability of LLTTs as a baseline group, particularly in older subjects. The fall in cardiovascular mortality risk in the heavy drinkers may well point to the "hard core" of stable heavy drinkers at Q92 who eventually succumb to non-cardiovascular causes of death, reflected in their increased relative risk of total mortality at Q92.

Table 5. Relative risk for cardiovascular and total mortality at Q5 and Q92 adjusted for age, smoking, social class, BMI and pre-existing disease/medication.

| Alcohol intake | CVD | | Total | |
| --- | --- | --- | --- | --- |
| | (Q5) | (Q92) | (Q5) | (Q92) |
| TT | 0.92 | 1.60* | 1.02 | 1.22 |
| EX | 1.38* | 1.76* | 1.28 | 1.45* |
| Occ | 1.00 | 1.00 | 1.00 | 1.00 |
| Light | 0.84 | 0.91 | 0.93 | 0.82 |
| Moderate | 0.95 | 0.97 | 1.06 | 0.94 |
| Heavy | 1.09 | 0.73 | 1.02 | 1.53* |

* = p<0.05

## Conclusions

Light drinkers, particularly stable light drinkers, have life style characteristics and patterns of ill health and medication which are markedly advantageous compared to all other alcohol intake categories. Non-drinkers, on the other hand, include a significant number of those who have been regular drinkers in the past (light, moderate, or heavy). Their characteristics, particularly if they are recent ex-drinkers, are the least advantageous of any alcohol intake category and their proportion in relation to all non-drinkers, increases with age. It is thus not surprising that what is remarkably consistent in studies of alcohol and outcomes is that light drinkers do well and non-drinkers do badly. Adjustments for favorable and unfavorable characteristics almost always result in light drinkers showing lower relative risks for mortality than other groups. In addition, there are plausible mechanisms to account for the benefits of alcohol on CHD specifically. However, whether adjustments can adequately take into account all the differences between alcohol intake categories, seems uncertain and the magnitude of the protective effect of regular light drinking may be exaggerated by the choice of baseline and by residual confounding.

## Acknowledgments

The British Regional Heart Study is supported by the British Heart Foundation and the UK Department of Health.

## References

1.    Wannamethee G, Shaper AG, Whincup PH, Walker M. Low serum total cholesterol concentration and mortality in middle-aged British men. BMJ 1985;311:409-13.
2.    Wannamethee G, Shaper AG. Body weight and mortality in middle-aged British men: Impact of smoking. BMJ 1989;299:1497-1502.
3.    Wannamethee G, Shaper AG. Changes in drinking habits in middle-aged British men. J Roy Coll Gen Pract 1988;38:440-42.
4.    Wannamethee G, Shaper AG. Men who do not drink: A report from the British Regional Heart Study. Int J Epidemiol 1988;17:307-16.
5.    Shaper AG, Wannamethee SG. The J-shaped curve and changes in drinking habit. In: Chadwick DJ, Goode JA, editors. Alcohol and cardiovascular diseases. Novartis Foundation Symposium No.216. Chichester, UK: John Wiley & Sons, 1998:173-92.
6.    Wannamethee SG, Shaper AG. Lifelong teetotallers, ex-drinkers and drinkers: Mortality and the incidence of coronary heart disease events in middle-aged British men. Int J Epidemiol 1997;26:523-31.

Additional reference: Wannamethee SG, Shaper AG. Type of alcoholic drink and risk of major coronary heart disease events and all cause mortality. Am J Public Health 1999;89:685-90.

ADVERSE CARDIOVASCULAR EFFECTS OF ALCOHOL

Markku Kupari

## Introduction

The effects of alcohol on the structure and function of the circulatory organs are tightly consumption-related. Used in moderation, alcohol may have a favorable overall influence on the cardiovascular health, while chronic heavy drinking predisposes to heart muscle disease, arrhythmias, sudden death, hypertension and cerebrovascular accidents.

## Alcohol and Cardiac Function

ACUTE EFFECTS

Alcohol acutely impairs myocardial contractions. This negative inotropic effect can be detected *in vitro* at concentrations of ethanol as low as 2-4 mmol/l [1]. Acute reductions in both intracellular calcium transients and calcium sensitivity of the contractile myofilaments are involved [2]. The ultimate mechanism, however, is alcohol's influence on the biological membranes. Due to high lipid- and water-solubility, alcohol easily penetrates and permeates the phospholipid bilayers altering the fluidity of the membranes as well as the function of ion channels traversing the membrane. Experimental studies with different alcohols have shown that the longer the carbon side chain of the molecule is, a direct determinant of lipid solubility, the stronger is the acute negative inotropic effect [3].

Moving from isolated myocardial strips to an intact human body, the negative inotropic effect is counteracted and modified by a number of other effects of alcohol like acute sympatho-adrenergic stimulation, vasodilation and increased diuresis [4]. The net change in left ventricular function depends on the dose of alcohol, on the postintake timing of the measurements and on the function of the autonomic nervous system, whether it is intact or partially or fully blocked. Importantly, left ventricular systolic function may actually be stimulated early postalcohol, due to sympatho-adrenergic excitation and vasodilation, despite negative inotropy [5]. However, the acute impairment of contractility becomes apparent *in vivo*, too, when cardiac function is studied during autonomic blockade [6] or using sensitive and load-independent means like end-systolic pressure-volume relations [7]. Lang and associates measured left ventricular end-systolic pressure-diameter slope by echocardiography in healthy subjects ingesting 1.15 g of alcohol per kg body

113

R. Paoletti et al. (eds.), Moderate Alcohol Consumption and Cardiovascular Disease, 113–120.
© 2000 Kluwer Academic Publishers and Fondazione Giovanni Lorenzini. Printed in the Netherlands.

weight. They found a consistent decrease in the steepness of the slope, indicating depressed contractility, even though left ventricular pump function remained largely unaltered [7]. The role of the acute vasodilatory and diuretic actions of alcohol is well seen in heart failure. Greenberg et al. gave 0.9 g/kg alcohol to patients with severe congestive heart failure and found that peripheral arterial resistance and pulmonary wedge pressure were markedly decreased without any change in cardiac pumping capacity [8]. Thus, despite direct negative inotropy, the net short-term influence of alcohol in heart failure was beneficial rather than detrimental, owing to the effects of alcohol on cardiac loading conditions. It must be recognized, however, that these data tell nothing about the consequences of regular modest use of alcohol in heart failure.

Inherited (or drug-related) abnormalities in alcohol metabolism can modify the acute effects of alcohol intake on the heart and circulation [9,10]. Genetically deficient acetaldehyde dehydrogenase activity is a common trait among Orientals and leads to acetaldehyde accumulation with facial flushing after alcohol intake ("Oriental flushers"). Figure 1 shows the effect of a small dose of alcohol on hemodynamics in two groups of Japanese men (flushers and nonflushers by history) compared with Finnish men. There is no question that the intensity of cardiac stimulation is sufficient to produce adverse consequences in susceptible people with cardiac disease, no matter whether acetaldehyde accumulates due to an inherited or a drug-induced inhibition acetaldehyde dehydrogenase.

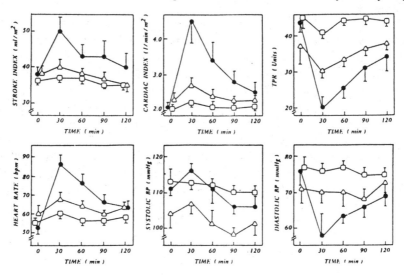

Figure 1. Hemodynamic effect of oral intake of alcohol, 0.5 g/kg body weight, in Japanese male flushers (closed circles, n = 5), Japanese male nonflushers (open triangles, n = 4) and Finnish men (open squares, n = 10). In Japanese men with a history of postalcohol flush, blood acetaldehyde rose to a mean of 43 umol/l after alcohol. In the other Japanese and Finnish subjects, acetaldehyde was not detected in blood postalcohol. BP = blood pressure, TPR = total peripheral resistance

CHRONIC EFFECTS IN THE GENERAL POPULATION

There exist very little data on the effects of long-term alcohol consumption on left ventricular function in the general population with a wide range of drinking habits. In a study of a random sample of120 persons aged 36-37 years, the participants recorded their daily alcohol use for a 3-month period and underwent thereafter a cardiac ultrasound study. Left ventricular fractional shortening showed a statistically significant inverse association with daily alcohol dose suggesting a minor yet detectable cardiodepression from habitual drinking [11]. In this study, left ventricular mass was unrelated to daily alcohol consumption, but in the Framingham study, which involved a much larger population sample, left ventricular mass was directly and independently related to daily alcohol dose, particularly in men [12].

ALCOHOLIC HEART MUSCLE DISEASE

Alcoholic heart muscle disease results from years of heavy drinking. Studies have shown that acoholics frequently have left ventricular hypertrophy and impairment of diastolic function without any symptoms aside perhaps from a propensity to arrhythmias [13,14] About one in three alcoholics may have a slight dilatation of the left ventricle with impairment of systolic function [15,16], but clinically evident congestive dilated cardiomyopathy is seen in only 1 to 3% of alcoholics. Though small at first sight, this prevalence figure is still 100 times the prevalence of dilated cardiomyopathy in the general population.
       The detailed pathogenesis of alcohol-induced heart muscle injury is still not established [17]. Table 1 lists some of the proposed mechanisms. The relation of heart muscle involvement to the quantity of alcohol consumption also remains unknown in detail. Although some studies suggest a linear association of left ventricular dysfunction and hypertrophy with the estimated total lifetime alcohol consumption [15,16], other works have been unable to expose any simple dose-injury relation for the effects of heavy drinking on the heart [18,19]. It is possible that in order to produce clinically evident dilated cardiomyopathy alcohol-induced cardiotoxicity must be combined either with individual (inherited) sensitivity or with other noxious effects on the myocardium like hypertension, viral infections, or dietary factors. The epidemic of cobalt-beer cardiomyopathy serves an example thereof [20].

**Alcohol and Arrhythmias**

Chest palpitation is a common symptom after alcohol intake, but in light to moderate drinkers alcohol has little real influence on cardiac rhythm aside from acceleration of the contraction rate. While uncontrolled electrophysiologic studies have shown an inconsistent prolongation of intracardiac conduction in nonalcoholic cardiac patients [21], more clinically oriented studies using Holter monitoring have shown only varying changes in the number of ectopic beats without significant arrhythmias [22]. Chronic heavy drinking, however, seems to increase the vulnerability to arrhythmias. The Holiday Heart syndrome was described as clustering of atrial arrhythmias after periods of heavy drinking in alcoholics [23]. The original idea has survived although later studies have suggested that the phenomenon may be apparent rather than real and due to reduced number of arrhythmias in nonheavy drinkers during weekends and holidays [24]. Controlled studies of consecutive admissions for supraventricular arrhythmias have shown that new-onset idiopathic atrial fibrillation frequently is associated with higher than ordinary alcohol consumption and that recurrent atrial fibrillation is associated with problem drinking particularly in men [25,26]. Electrophysiologic studies have revealed that acute alcohol intake can facilitate the induction of both atrial and ventricular tachyarrhythmias in selected alcoholic persons [27,28]. In a follow-up of more than 100,000 individuals participating in the Kaiser-Permanente program, the combined risk of all atrial tachyarrhythmias in people who consumed more than 6 drinks/day was more than double the risk of individuals consuming less than one drink/day [29].

Table 1. Possible Mechanisms of Alcohol-Induced Chronic Myocardial Toxicity

| |
|---|
| Toxic influence of fatty acyl ethyl esters |
| Free radical-related injury |
| Increased intracellular calcium concentration |
| Inhibition of protein synthesis |
| Toxic and immunologic effects of acetaldehyde and acetaldehyde-protein adducts. |

Heavy drinking not only increases the propensity to arrhythmias but also associates with the risk of sudden cardiac death [30]. The British Regional Heart Study [31] followed 7,735 men aged 40-59 years for an 8-year period. Men in the highest drinking category (> 6 drinks/day) had an increased risk of sudden cardiac death compared with men who drank less or not at all; the relative risk was 1.73 (95% confidence interval, 1.06-2.86) after adjustment for age, social class, and smoking. The role of alcohol was particularly evident in older men and in men without pre-existing ischemic heart disease. Prospective studies in Scandinavia have also shown that sudden cardiac death is associated with history of alcohol consumption [32] and with registrations for alcohol intemperance [33].

Table 2 lists the candidate mechanisms underlying the risk of cardiac arrhythmias and sudden death in alcoholics. Subclinical heart muscle disease which patchy fibrosis certainly can predispose to re-entry tachyarrhythmias. Abnormal repolarization with prolonged QT-interval and impaired vagal control of cardiac rate have both been associated with increased mortality in alcoholics [34,35] QT-dispersion, however, has not been increased in alcoholics relative to healthy persons [34]. Acute alcohol intake has been shown to reduce heart rate variability in healthy persons and patients with ischemic heart disease alike [36,37]. There also exists evidence that acute alcohol ingestion may blunt the sensitivity of the baroreflex arc, but definitive studies are lacking [36].

Table 2. Possible Arrhythmogenic Mechanisms of Alcohol-Related Cardiac Arrhythmias and Sudden Death

| |
| --- |
| Subclinical heart muscle injury |
| Sympatho-adrenergic stimulation |
| Prolongation of ventricular depolarization |
| Reduced vagal control of heart rate |
| Electrolyte disturbances |
| Worsening of sleep apnea |
| Worsening of myocardial ischemia |

**Hypertension and Cerebrovascular Accidents**

Numerous studies with different designs have confirmed an association between blood pressure and alcohol consumption and the causal role of alcohol has been proved beyond any reasonable doubt [38]. According to current knowledge, habitual use of more than 30 g/day increases blood pressure in a linear dose-dependent manner. Heavy drinkers have on average 8 to 10 mmHg higher systolic blood pressure and 2 to 6 mmHg higher diastolic blood pressure than the remaining population. As a rule of thumb, above 30 g/day of habitual alcohol intake an increment of 10 g/day increases systolic and diastolic blood pressure by 1-2 mmHg and 1 mmHg, respectively [37]. The prevalence of hypertension (> 160/90 mmHg) is elevated 1.6 to 4 times in heavy drinkers, and alcohol-related high blood pressure may explain from 5% to 11% of "essential" hypertension in men [39,40]. The mechanism of alcohol-related hypertension is not established. Sympatho-adrenergic overactivity is a candidate as are baroreceptor dysfunction, activation of the renin-angiotensin-aldosterone system, vascular endothelial dysfunction, and increased calcium concentration in the smooth muscle cells of the arterial walls. Important from the clinical standpoint, intervention studies have consistently demonstrated that blood pressure decreases as heavy drinkers abstain or restrict their alcohol intake [37,41].

Alcohol-related increase in blood pressure is probably one of the mechanisms underlying the elevated risk of cerebrovascular accidents in heavy drinkers [42]. It is generally agreed that heavy use of alcohol doubles the risk of intracerebral hemorrhage and also increases the risk of ischemic stroke and subarachnoidal hemorrhage. In addition to fluctuation of blood pressure, alcohol-induced changes in hemostatic and fibrinolytic factors [43] may play a role. However, the association between stroke and alcohol is very complex in that light-to-moderate consumption may in fact have a protective effect. These questions are discussed more in depth in a separate chapter of this book.

## Conclusions

The adverse cardiovascular effects of alcohol include myocardial injury which usually is asymptomatic but may lead to congestive dilated cardiomyopathy, a propensity to arrhythmias and sudden death, increased blood pressure, and increased risk of all subtypes of stroke. Reassuringly, however, these problems associate with heavy drinking only. A small and clinically insignificant negative inotropic effect aside, drinking in moderation is not bad for anybody's heart or circulation save perhaps people with abnormal alcohol metabolism.

## References

1.      Mason DT, Spann JF, Miller RR, Lee G, Arbogast R, Segel LD. Effects of acute ethanol exposure on the contractile state of normal and failing cat papillary muscles. Eur J Cardiol 1978;7:311-15.
2.      Danziger RS. Sakai M. Capogrossi MC. Spurgeon HA. Hansford RG. Lakatta EG. Ethanol acutely and reversibly suppresses excitation-contraction coupling in cardiac myocytes. Circulation Res 1991;68:1160-68.
3.      Nakano J, Moore SE. Effect of different alcohols on the contractile force of the isolated guinea-pig myocardium. Eur J Pharmacol 1972;20:266-301.
4.      Kupari M. Acute cardiovascular effects of ethanol. A controlled non-invasive study. Br Heart J 1983;49:174-80.
5.      Kupari M, Heikkilä J, Tolppanen E-M, Nieminen MS, Ylikahri R. Acute effects of alcohol, beta-blockade and their combination on left ventricular function and hemodynamics in normal man. Eur Heart J 1983;4:463-71.
6.      Child JS, Kovick RB, Levisman JA, Pearce ML, Cardiac effects of acute ethanol ingestion unmasked by autonomic blockade. Circulation 1979;59:120-25.
7.      Lang RM, Borow KM, Neumann A, Feldman T. Adverse cardiac effects of alcohol in young adults. Ann Intern Med 1985;102:742-47.
8.      Greenberg BH, Schutz R, Grunkemeier GL, Griswold H. Acute effects of alcohol in patients with congestive heart failure. Ann Intern Med 1982;97:171-75.
9.      Kupari M, Lindros K, Hillbom M, Heikkilä J, Ylikahri R. Acute cardiovascular effects of acetaldehyde accumulation after ethanol ingestion: their modification by beta-adrenergic blockade and alcohol dehydrogenase inhibition. Alcoholism: Clin Exp Res 1983;7:283-88.
10.     Kupari M, Eriksson CJP, Heikkilä J, Ylikahri R. Alcohol and the heart: Intense hemodynamic changes associated with alcohol flush in Orientals. Acta Med Scand 1983; 213:91-98.
11.     Kupari M, Koskinen P. Relation of left ventricular function to habitual alcohol consumption in a population sample. Am J Cardiol 1993;72:1418-24.
12.     Manolio TA, Levy D, Garrison RJ, Castelli WP, Kannel WB. Relation of alcohol intake

to left ventricular mass: The Framingham Study. J Am Coll Cardiol 1991;17:717-21.

13. Silberbauer K, Juhasz M, Ohrenberger G, Hess C. Noninvasive assessment of left ventricular diastolic function by pulsed Doppler echocardiography in young alcoholics. Cardiology 1988;75:431-39.

14. Kupari M, Koskinen P, Suokas A, Ventilä M. Left ventricular filling impairment in asymptomatic chronic alcoholics. Am J Cardiol 1990;66:1473-77.

15. Urbano-Marquez A, Estruch R, Navarro-Lopez F, Grau JM, Mont L, Rubin E. The effects of alcoholism on skeletal and cardiac muscle. N Engl J Med. 1989;320:409-415.

16. Urbano-Marquez A, Estruch R, Fernandez-Sola J, Nicolas JM, Pare JC, Rubin E: The greater risk of alcoholic cardiomyopathy and myopathy in women compared with men. JAMA 1995;274:149-54.

17. Richardson PJ, Patel VB, Preedy VR. Alcohol and the myocardium. Novartis Foundation Symposium 1998;216:35-45.

18. Mathews EC, Gardin JM, Henry WL, et al. Echocardiographic abnormalities in chronic alcoholics with and without congestive heart failure. Am J Cardiol 1981;47:570-78.

19. Kupari M, Koskinen P, Suokas A. Left ventricular size, mass and function in relation to the duration and quantity of heavy drinking in alcoholics. Am J Cardiol 1991;67:274-79.

20. Alexander CS. Cobalt and the heart. Ann Intern Med 1969;70:411-13.

21. Gould L, Reddy CVR, Becker W, Oh K-C, Kim SG. Electrophysiologic properties of alcohol in man. J Electrocardiol 1978;11:219-26.

22. Kentala E, Luurila O, Salaspuro M. Effects of alcohol ingestion on cardiac rhythm in patients with ischemia heart disease. Ann Clin Res 1976;8:408-14.

23. Ettinger PO, Wu CF, DeLaCruz C, Weisse AB, Ahmed SS, Regan TJ. Arrhythmias and the "Holiday Heart": Alcohol-associated cardiac rhythm disorders. Am Heart J 1978;95: 555-62.

24. Kupari M, Koskinen P. Time of onset of supraventricular tachyarrhythmia in relation to alcohol consumption. Am J Cardiol 1991;67:718-22.

25. Koskinen P, Kupari M, Leinonen H, Luomanmäki K. Alcohol and new-onset atrial fibrillation: A case-control study of a current series. Br Heart J 1987;57:468-73.

26. Koskinen P, Kupari M, Leinonen H. Role of alcohol in recurrences of atrial fibrillation in patients of working age. Am J Cardiol 1990;66:954-5.

27. Greenspon AJ, Schaal SF. The "holiday heart": Electrophysiologic studies of alcohol effects in alcoholics. Ann Intern Med 1983;98:135-39.

28. Greenspon AJ, Stang JM, Lewis RP, Schaal SF. Provocation of ventricular tachycardia after consumption of alcohol. N Engl J Med 1979;301: 049-50.

29. Cohen EJ, Klatsky AL, Armstrong MA. Alcohol use and supraventricular arrhythmia. Am J Cardiol 1988;62:971-73.

30. Kupari M, Koskinen P. Alcohol, cardiac arrhythmias and sudden death. Novartis Foundation Symposium 1998;216:68-85.

31. Wannamethee G, Shaper AG. Alcohol and sudden cardiac death. Br Heart J 1992;68:443-48.

32. Suhonen O, Aromaa A, Reunanen A, Knekt P. Alcohol consumption and sudden cardiac death in middle-aged Finnish men. Acta Med Scand 1987;221:335-41.

33. Lithell H, Åberg H, Selinus I, Hedstrand H. Alcohol intemperance and sudden death. Br Med J 1987;294:1456-58.

34. Day CP, James OF, Butler TJ, Campbell RW. QT prolongation and sudden cardiac death

in alcoholics with liver disease. Lancet 1993;341:1423-28.

35.    Johnson RH, Robinson BJ. Mortality in chronic alcoholics. J Neurol Neurosurg Psychiatry 1988;51:476-80.

36.    Koskinen P, Virolainen J, Kupari M. Acute alcohol intake decreases short-term heart rate variability in healthy subjects. Clin Science 1994;87:225-30.

37.    Rossinen J, Viitasalo M, Partanen J, Koskinen P, Kupari M, Nieminen MS. Effects of acute alcohol ingestion on heart rate variability in patients with documented coronary artery disease. Am J Cardiol 1997;79:487-91.

38.    Keil U, Liese A, Filipiak B, Swales JD, Grobbee DE. Alcohol, blood pressure and hypertension. Novartis Foundation Symposium 1998;216:125-51.

39.    Keil U, Chambless L, Remmers A. Alcohol and blood pressure: results from the Lubeck Blood Pressure Study. Prev Med 1989;18:1-10.

40.    MacMahon SW, Blacket RB, MacDonald GJ, Hall W. Obesity, alcohol consumption and blood pressure in Australian men and women. The National Heart Foundation of Australia Risk Factor Prevalence Study. J Hypertension 1984;2:85-91.

41.    Potter JF, Beevers DG. Pressor effect f alcohol in hypertension. Lancet 1984;1:119-22.

42.    Hillbom M, Juvela S, Karttunen V. Mechanisms of alcohol-related strokes. Novartis Foundation Symposium 1998;216:193-207.

43.    Hendriks HJF, van der Graag MS. Alcohol, coagulation and fibrinolysis. Novartis Foundation Symposium 1998;216:111-24.

# BEER, WINE, SPIRITS, AND CARDIOVASCULAR DISEASE

Morten Grønbæk

## Introduction

Many epidemiological studies have described a U-shaped relation between alcohol intake and all-cause mortality [1-4]. Most researchers attribute the "U" to a combination of beneficial and harmful effects of ethanol itself. It has, on the other hand, been explained as an artefact due to misclassification or confounding [5]. Most of the studies of the effect of total alcohol intake have found that the descending leg of the curve mainly is attributable to death from cardiovascular disease [6,7].

The relation between alcohol and cardiovascular disease has been shown to be influenced by age and cardiovascular risk factor status [3]. The question whether it is also influenced by which type of beverage drunk will be addressed in this paper.

## Correlational Studies

Until recently, most studies addressed the effect of the three beverages (beer, wine, and spirits) taken together as ethanol. Studies of the correlation between wine intake per capita in different countries and incidence of ischemic heart disease gave rise to the hypothesis that there is a more beneficial effect of wine than of beer and spirits. St. Leger et al., Renaud et al., and later Criqui et al. found an inverse relation between incidence rates of ischemic heart disease and wine consumption in different countries, but no such relation for the other types of beverages [8-10].

## Prospective Cohort Studies

Several population studies of the effect of alcohol on cardiovascular disease mortality have addressed the question of different effects of the different types of beverages. The studies have in common that they mention their finding: "no significant difference," "a trend towards a stronger effect of beer," etc. in a few sentences during a paper itself devoted to the analysis of effect of alcohol on coronary heart disease or mortality. It is, therefore, quite difficult to extract from the papers, the distribution of intake of the different beverages, and how the authors reached their conclusions. Rimm et al. include in a recent review ten

121

R. Paoletti et al. (eds.), Moderate Alcohol Consumption and Cardiovascular Disease, 121–126.
© 2000 Kluwer Academic Publishers and Fondazione Giovanni Lorenzini. Printed in the Netherlands.

prospective population studies, of which three did not analyze the effect of all three types of alcoholic beverages because of a negligible consumption of one or two of them [11]. The analysis in two other studies did not take into account intake of the other types of beverages. Of the remaining five studies, four supported a greater beneficial effect of wine although with different methodological and statistical strength.

A recent study from Great Britain showed that all-cause mortality and cardiovascular disease was influenced by type of beverage drunk. Hence, Wannamethee and Shaper found that drinkers of wine were at a lower risk of death from cardiovascular disease than drinkers of beer and spirits [12].

The question of effect of the different types of alcoholic drinks on cardiovascular disease mortality can be approached in two different ways: 1) is it alcohol or another substance, or 2) is it alcohol and another substance which implies the beneficial effect. In their review, Rimm et al. used the first approach [11]. It was shown that the U-shaped relation between alcohol intake and cardiovascular disease mortality persisted in populations with very different drinking patterns, such as wine drinkers in Italy and beer drinkers on Hawaii. Hence, the lower risk of morbidity and mortality from cardiovascular disease among drinkers of a small dose of ethanol is a consistent finding.

The second approach, to answer the question whether other substances than ethanol have an additional beneficial effect, a significant intake of all three types of beverages in the particular population examined, is needed.

### Results from The Copenhagen City Heart Study

In the Copenhagen City Heart Study, wine drinkers experienced a significantly lower mortality from all causes as well as from cardiovascular disease than those who drank no wine (Table 1).

In these analyses variables for beer, wine, and spirits are introduced in the Poisson models. The reference group (relative risk=1.00) therefore differed from type to type. Even though patients taking disulfiram and dipsomanic patients were excluded from the analysis, these differences in reference groups may affect the interpretation of the results. Further, one would expect that the recognized effect of ethanol itself would imply an effect modification of drinking one type of alcohol on drinking the other on mortality. On the other hand, the influence of type of beverage on mortality was, in the range of intake from none to 3-5 drinks per day, statistically independent of each other, and persisted throughout the twelve years of follow-up [13].

### Different Explanations to the Findings from Prospective Cohort Studies

The reasons for the differences in cardiovascular mortality among wine, beer, and spirits drinkers may either be cardioprotective factors in wine apart from ethanol or they maybe due to differences among different traits between wine, beer, and spirits drinkers.

Table 1. Relative risk of death (95% confidence limits) from all causes and from cardiovascular disease as a function of reported intake of alcoholic beverages, The Copenhagen City Heart Study [13].

|  | Beer intake | Wine intake | Spirits intake |
|---|---|---|---|
| **Death from all causes** | | | |
| Never | 1.00 (reference) | 1.00 (reference) | 1.00 (reference) |
| Monthly | 0.81 (0.73-0.91) | 0.77 (0.71-0.85) | 0.86 (0.78-0.95) |
| Weekly | 0.96 (0.86-1.07) | 0.64 (0.56-0.73) | 0.99 (0.88-1.12) |
| Daily, 1-2 | 0.88 (0.78-0.99) | 0.61 (0.49-0.76) | 0.98 (0.84-1.14) |
| Daily, 3-5 | 0.95 (0.83-1.09) | 0.51 (0.32-0.81) | 1.34 (1.05-1.71) |
| **Death from cardiovascular disease** | | | |
| Never | 1.00 (reference) | 1.00 (reference) | 1.00 (reference) |
| Monthly | 0.79 (0.69-0.91) | 0.69 (0.62-0.77) | 0.95 (0.85-1.06) |
| Weekly | 0.87 (0.75-0.99) | 0.53 (0.45-0.63) | 1.08 (0.93-1.26) |
| Daily, 1-2 | 0.79 (0.68-0.91) | 0.47 (0.35-0.62) | 1.16 (0.98-1.39) |
| Daily, 3-5 | 0.72 (0.61-0.88) | 0.44 (0.24-0.80) | 1.35 (1.00-1-83) |

## Substances in Wine?

In the Copenhagen City Heart Study we found that the risk functions for all of the three beverages show a small decrease in risk of dying for monthly drinkers as compared to never-drinkers. This decrease may reflect the beneficial effect of ethanol itself on mortality. The increasing risk function for increasing spirits intake may then reflect the hazardous effects of ethanol. While the continuing decrease in mortality may reflect the effect of factors in wine other than ethanol. These beneficial factors seem to overrule the hazardous effects of ethanol in wine in the range of intake investigated. Or these factors act beneficially in cooperation with ethanol in wine.

The results thus strongly suggest that, in addition to the common effect of ethanol, there are, within the studied range of drinking, different factors influencing health in the three types of beverages. Specifically, the results raise the question of what might be the protective agent in wine or the damaging factors in beer and spirits apart from ethanol? During the last couple of years other explanations of the possible biological mechanisms of wine have been found. The decreased cardio- and cerebrovascular disease mortality, also among beer drinkers, may reflect a common effect of ethanol on high density lipoprotein or fibrinolytic factors [14-18]. Further, an inverse relation has been found between alcohol intake and platelet aggregability, and, in agreement with our results, this has been shown to be even stronger for wine [16,18]. Our finding that only wine drinking clearly reduces both risk of dying from cardio- and cerebrovascular disease, and risk of dying from other causes, may suggest that other more broadly acting factors in wine are involved. Some of which are to be dealt with elsewhere in this supplement.

Flavonoids such as quercetin, rutin, catechin, and epicatechin are present in red wine, responsible for the color of the wine. These compounds *in vitro* have been found to inhibit eicosanoid synthesis and platelet aggregation [19,20]. Frankel et al. found flavonoids to be 10-20 times as potent as vitamin $E_1$ and found an inhibition of low density lipoprotein oxidation in humans by these phenolic substances, which was confirmed by Kondo et al. [15]. Hertog et al. found a preventive effect of dietary flavonoids on risk of developing ischemic heart disease [21].

## Confounders

Our finding, that moderate wine drinkers show a decrease in mortality larger than that found among moderate drinkers of beer and spirits, may be confounded by various genetic or other life-style related factors. Among nonwine drinkers 67% were current smokers, while 54% of wine drinkers were current smokers. Further, a larger proportion of wine drinkers belonged to the higher social class, as indicated by income and educational levels. These factors were thoroughly controlled for in all analyses [13]. However, a recent study from Denmark has shown that wine drinkers have a healthier diet than beer or spirits drinkers. Hence, wine drinkers had a much more frequent intake of both vegetables, fruits, fish, and olive oil (Mediterranean diet) than beer or spirits drinkers [22]. Further, it has been found in another cross-sectional study from Copenhagen, that wine drinkers are at a better self-reported health than beer or spirits drinkers (Table 2). No data on dietary habits among the subjects were available, and wine intake may be strongly associated with a healthy Mediterranean diet. It must be kept in mind that to explain the observed effect, the diet or another life-style factor itself, apart from being strongly associated with wine intake, should have a very significant effect on longevity.

## Conclusion

Drinkers of any type of alcoholic beverages have lower mortality due to cardiovascular disease than abstainers. The question whether substances other than alcohol in one or two of the beverages has an effect additional to that of ethanol has been sparsely studied. The few studies including a sufficient number of cases and a sufficient range of intake of the three types of beverages suggest that wine has those properties with regard to mortality from cardiovascular disease. The findings may be confounded by diet and other life-style factors, but are supported by pertinent experimental, clinical, and correlational studies.

Table 2. Is intake of type of beverage associated with self-reported subjective health? Adjusted odds ratios for suboptimal health, according to intake of different types of alcoholic beverages. From Grønbæk et al. [23].

| | Type specific alcohol intake, drinks per week | | | |
|---|---|---|---|---|
| | 0 | 1-2 | 3-5 | more than 5 |
| Beer | 1.0 (-) | 0.9 (0.7-1.1) | 1.4 (1.0-1.9) | 1.7 (1.2-2.5) |
| Wine | 1.0 (-) | 0.7 (0.6-0.9) | 0.7 (0.5-0.9) | 1.1 (0.6-2.2) |
| Spirits | 1.0 (-) | 0.9 (0.8-1.3) | 1.7 (1.1-2.8) | 2.7 (1.1-6.5) |

Adjusted for age, sex, intake of other types of alcoholic beverages, presence of chronic disease, educational level, body mass index, smoking habits, level of physical activity, and social networks. From Journal of Epidemiology and Community Health 1999;53:721-24.

## References

1.   Boffetta P, Garfinkel L. Alcohol drinking and mortality among men enrolled in an American cancer society prospective study. Epidemiology 1990;1:342-48.
2.   Marmot MG, Rose G, Shipley MJ, Thomas BJ. Alcohol and mortality: a U-shaped curve. Lancet 1981;March 14:580-83.
3.   Fuchs CS, Stampfer MJ, Colditz GA, et al. Alcohol consumption and mortality among women. N Engl J Med 1995;332:1245-50.
4.   Grønbæk M, Deis a, Sørensen TIA, et al. Influence of sex, age, body mass index, and smoking on alcohol and mortality. Br Med J 1994;308:302-6.
5.   Shaper AG, Wannamethee G, Walker M. Alcohol and mortality in British men: Explaining the U-shaped curve. Lancet 1988;2:1267-73.
6.   Stampfer MJ, Golditz GA, Willett WC, Speizer FE, Hennekens CH. a prospective study of moderate alcohol consumption and the risk of coronary disease and stroke in women. N Engl J Med 1988;319:267-73.
7.   Rimm EB, Giovannucci EL, Willett WC, et al. Prospective study of alcohol consumption and risk of coronary disease in men. Lancet 1991;338:464-68.
8.   Criqui MH, Rigel BL. Does diet or alcohol explain the French paradox? Lancet 1994; 344:1719-23.
9.   St Leger AS, Cochrane AL, Moore F. Factors associated with cardiac mortality in developed countries with particular reference to the consumption of wine. Lancet 1979;i:1017-20.
10.  Renaud S, de Lorgeril M. Wine, alcohol, platelets, and the French paradox for coronary heart disease. Lancet 1992;39:1523-26.
11.  Rimm EB, Klatsky A, Grobbee D, Stampfer MJ. Review of moderate alcohol consumption and reduced risk of coronary heart disease: is the effect due to beer, wine or spirits? Br Med J 1996;312:731-36.

12.     Wannamethee SG, Shaper AG. Type of alcoholic drink and risk of major coronary heart disease events and all-cause mortality. Am J Public Health 1999;89:685-90.

13.     Grønbæk M, Deis A, Sørensen TIA, Becker U, Schnohr P, Jensen G. Mortality associated with moderate intake of wine, beer, or spirits. Br Med J 1995;310:1165-69.

14.     Frankel EN, Kanner J, German JB, Parks E, Kinsella JE. Inhibition of oxidation of human low-density lipoprotein by phenolic substances in red wine. Lancet 1993;341: 454-57.

15.     Kondo K, Matsumoto A, Kurata H, Tanahashi H, Koda H, Amachi T. Inhibition of oxidation of low-density lipoprotein with red wine. Lancet 1994;344:1152-52.

16.     Struck M, Watkins T, Tomeo A, Halley J, Bierenboum M. Effect of red and white wine on serum lipids, platelet aggregation, oxidation products and antioxidants: A preliminary report. Nutr Research 1994;14:1811-19.

17.     Fuhrman B, Lavy A, Aviram M. Consumption of red wine with meals reduces the susceptibility of human plasma and low-density lipoprotein to lipid peroxidation.Am J Clin Nutr 1995;61:549-54.

18.     Ruf J-C, Berger JL, Renaud S. Platelet rebound effect of alcohol withdrawal and wine drinking in rats - relation to tannins and lipid peroxidation. Arterioscler Thromb Vasc Biol 1995;15:140-44.

19.     Goldberg DM. Does wine work? Clin Chem 1995;41:14-16.

20.     Whitehead TP, Robinson D, Allaway S, Syms J, Hale A. Effect of red wine ingestion on the antioxidant capacity of serum. Clin Chem 1995;41:32-35.

21.     Hertog MGL, Feskens EJM, Hollman PCH, Katan MK, Kromhout D. Dietary antioxidant flavonoids and risk of coronary heart disease: The Zutphen Elderly Study. Lancet 1993; 342:1007-11.

22.     Tjønneland A, Grønbæk M, Stripp C, Overvad K. Wine intake and diet in a random sample of 48763 Danish men and women. Am J Clin Nutr 1999;69:49-54.

23.     Grønbæk M, Mortensen EL, Mygind K, et al. Beer, wine, spirits and subjective health. J Epidemiol Community Health 1999:53:721-24.

# ALCOHOLIC BEVERAGES AND CARDIOVASCULAR DISEASE PROTECTION: THE EFFECT OF ALCOHOL OR OTHER COMPONENTS?

Eric Rimm

## Introduction

The inverse association between moderate alcohol consumption and lower risk of cardiovascular disease has been documented in many large observational studies from around the world. In general, moderate intake of alcohol in the form of beer, wine, or spirits reduces the risk of fatal and nonfatal coronary heart disease and ischemic stroke by approximately 25-40%. In recent years, results from studies in Denmark, France, and the United States have suggested that wine, specifically red wine, may be more beneficial than other alcohol-containing beverages; however, an equal number of studies from countries where red wine is not the alcoholic beverage of choice have found that beer or spirits are equally protective. Differences between studies may be attributed to differences in drinking patterns or other lifestyle traits such as diet or physical activity. The protection afforded by moderate alcohol consumption is due mainly to its effects on lipid levels and hemostatic factors; therefore, alcohol from any beverage choice, when consumed in moderation, will significantly decrease risk of cardiovascular disease.

Twenty-five years ago, Klatsky et al. [1] observed an inverse association between alcohol and coronary heart disease and later Barboriak et al. [2] found that moderate alcohol consumption was associated with reduced occlusive disease in patients with coronary angiography. These findings sparked a new era in alcohol research which focused on identifying the health effects (risks and benefits) associated with moderate alcohol consumption. The large body of evidence from epidemiological studies suggests that alcohol in moderation ($\leq$ 2 drinks/day for men and $\leq$1 drink/day for women) is associated with a lower risk of coronary heart disease, diabetes, and ischemic stroke. Because cardiovascular disease is the leading cause of death among men and women, results from large prospective studies of alcohol and all-cause mortality consistently find the lowest risk of death among moderate drinkers.

## Moderate Drinking

For many years the definition of moderate consumption has caused confusion and in some cases made it difficult to compare results across studies in the United States and in Europe.

*R. Paoletti et al. (eds.), Moderate Alcohol Consumption and Cardiovascular Disease, 127–132.*
© 2000 *Kluwer Academic Publishers and Fondazione Giovanni Lorenzini. Printed in the Netherlands.*

In the United Kingdom, moderation is defined as 21 units a week for men and 14 units a week for women; a unit is 10 g of alcohol. In the United States, the most recent dietary guidelines define moderate drinking as up to 2 drinks a day for men and 1 drink a day for women [3]. Because a 5-ounce glass of wine, a 12-ounce beer and a 1.5-ounce shot of 80 proof spirits have similar amounts of alcohol (approximately 12.5-14 grams), the type of beverage is not important when defining moderation. For the purposes of this review, I will consider consumption of alcohol up to 30 g/day as moderate.

Results of ecologic, case-control, and prospective studies published over the last 30 years consistently show that a moderate intake of alcohol in the form of beer, wine, or spirits reduces the risk of fatal and nonfatal coronary heart disease (CHD) by approximately 25-40%. Recent results from very large cohort studies which, in total, have followed over 1,000,000 subjects, confirm this association. In recent years, Moore and Pearson [4], Kannel [5], Veenstra [6], Marmot and Brummer [7], Poikolainen [8], Jackson and Beaglehole [9], Klatsky [10], and Rimm et al. [11,12] have produced extensive reviews and discussed the scientific evidence available. The wealth of information in this area is too substantial to describe in detail in this review, but specific studies which address the beverage-specific association between alcohol and cardiovascular disease are described below.

Several studies [10,11,13-25] have separately assessed consumption of wine, beer, and spirits and presented beverage-specific relative risks. From these studies it can be inferred that there is no clear evidence that one type of beverage is more protective than another. Recently, we summarized the available literature from ecologic, case-control, and cohort studies [11]. Although most ecological studies support the hypothesis that wine consumption is most beneficial, methodologic problems (e.g. unaccountable confounding, population rather individual assessment of consumption) limit their usefulness in drawing conclusions. Results from observational studies, in which individual consumption can be assessed in detail and linked directly to coronary heart disease, provide strong evidence that a substantial proportion of the benefits of wine, beer, or spirits is attributable to alcohol rather than other components of each drink.

Particular confidence can be given to the results of the most recent studies, which considered very large cohorts from several geographic locations. The studies below are highlighted because beverage choice (as well as lifestyle choices) in these populations vary dramatically, yet the underlying benefit of alcohol is relatively constant. For example, in a 7-year follow-up of 18,244 men from Shanghai, China, Yuan et al. [24] reported that men who consumed 1-28 drinks/week had a 36% reduction in ischemic heart disease mortality compared to abstainers. Of the 7,773 regular drinkers, 3,500 (45%) drank beer, 4,341 (56%) consumed wine, and 3,723 (48%) drank spirits. In the analysis of beverage choice and risk of noncancer mortality, moderate drinkers of beer, wine, or spirits achieved similar benefit. A very similar reduction in CHD (35%) was reported among women consuming 1-2 drinks/day (compared to abstainers) in the study of 85,709 women from the Nurses' Health Study [26]. Again, beverage choice was not important; benefits for coronary heart disease mortality were similar for all sources of ethanol. Other large studies from the United Kingdom, Japan, France, and Denmark have reported similar reductions in CHD among men and women. In addition to the size of these studies, the amazingly consistent findings across studies which have followed vastly different populations lends strong support to the hypothesis that alcohol in moderation lowers risk of coronary disease and that choice of beverage is not an important determinant of the magnitude of this reduction.

Although there is general consistency in the inverse association between average total alcohol consumption and risk of CVD, there are several studies which reported substantial benefit for only one specific beverage [18,20,23]. The association between beverage choice and lifestyle patterns may explain some of the dramatic differences found in epidemiologic studies of alcoholic beverage type and CHD [11,20]. In the Copenhagen City Heart Study, wine intake was strongly inversely associated with CHD mortality, beer had no association, and spirits were positively correlated with CHD mortality [20]. In a large cohort of 36,250 men from Eastern France, both beer and wine were associated with lower risk of cardiovascular death; the association for wine was stronger [23]. Although wine contains antioxidants [27,28], vasorelaxants [29], and stimulants to antiaggregatory mechanisms [30,31], other lifestyle factors correlated with wine consumption may be equally or more important [17]. In the Copenhagen City Heart Study cited above, data were not available on dietary practices, but in a separate large cohort study in Denmark, men and women who drank wine moderately had twice the intake of fruits and vegetables compared to their beer and spirits drinking counterparts [32]. This could explain that differences in beverage specific relative risks from the Copenhagen City Heart study. An additional benefit from a specific type of alcoholic beverage has not yet been satisfactorily established.

## Mechanisms

The effects of alcohol on the cardiovascular system are multifactorial, yet much of the benefit associated with moderate consumption is attributable to the increase in hign density lipoprotein (HDL) cholesterol and related apolipoproteins [12,33]. Among men and women Criqui et al. [34] reported a 50% reduction of the protective strength of the alcohol coefficient after the addition of HDL cholesterol to the model. Since this initial study, other case-control and cohort studies have reported that 45%-60% of the association between moderate alcohol consumption and risk of CHD is explained via the HDL cholesterol pathway [21,35-37].

In a recent meta-analysis of almost 40 metabolic studies of alcohol and HDL cholesterol [12], we estimated that a 30-gram intake of alcohol would increase HDL cholesterol by 3.99 mg/dl. If this increase in HDL cholesterol were projected to rates of CHD from the Framingham Heart Study, the overall effect of 30 g/day of alcohol would lower risk of CHD by 16.5%. Since most prospective analyses of moderate alcohol consumption and risk of CHD report a 25-40% reduction in risk, the projected 16.5% reduction in risk due solely to changes in HDL cholesterol is comparable in magnitude to the reduction suggested by the studies of Criqui and Langer discussed above [34,35].

In addition to the effects of alcohol on HDL cholesterol, other possible mechanisms are likely to play an important role. Decreased propensity of blood coagulation has been attributed to moderate alcohol consumption. Alcohol can lower fibrinogen [38] and inhibit platelet aggregation [12,39,40]. Recent evidence also suggests that independent of other known predictors of insulin, moderate alcohol consumption is associated with a decrease in fasting insulin levels [41,42] . All of these mechanisms are attributed to the effects of ethanol and generally not to other components of each beverage type. For example, in the meta-analysis of experimental studies of alcohol [12], regression models were fit using only studies which included beer, wine, spirits, or ethanol. The coefficients for alcohol from beer (b = 0.160; increase in HDL-C per gram of ethanol in beverage, n = 13 studies), wine (b = 0.132, n = 11), or spirits (b = 0.111, n = 4) were not significantly different from each other or from the coefficient among the remaining studies which provided either ethanol- or nonspecific-alcohol-containing beverages (b = 0.128, n = 8). Furthermore, the effects of ethanol on lipids, hemostatic factors, and insulin sensitivity are achievable at levels of moderate consumption, unlike reported antioxidant benefits of red wine which may require doses well above the definition of moderate consumption.

In conclusion, the currently available experimental, clinical and observational evidence strongly suggests that the association between alcohol consumption and cardiovascular disease (i.e. coronary heart disease and ischemic stroke) is causal. This causal association is more than likely due to the proven effects of ethanol on lipid and hemostatic factors rather than other components of alcoholic beverages. Further research is needed to help clarify the importance of drinking patterns, dietary interactions, and genetic susceptibility on reported associations between moderate consumption of beer, wine, or spirits and risk of cardiovascular disease.

# References

1.    Klatsky AL, Friedman GD, Siegelaub AB. Alcohol consumption before myocardial infarction. Results from the Kaiser-Permanente epidemiologic study of myocardial infarction. Ann Intern Med 1974;81:294-301.
2.    Barboriak JJ, Anderson AJ, Hoffmann RG. Interrelationship between coronary artery occlusion, high-density lipoprotein cholesterol, and alcohol intake. J Lab Clin Med 1979; 94:348-53.
3.    Food and Nutrition Board. Recommended Dietary Allowances, 10th revised edition. Washington, DC: National Academy of Sciences, 1989.
4.    Moore RD, Pearson TA. Moderate alcohol consumption and coronary artery disease: A review. Medicine 1986;65:242-67.
5.    Kannel WB. Alcohol and cardiovascular disease. Proc Nutr Soc 1988;47:99-110.
6.    Veenstra J. Moderate alcohol use and coronary heart disease: A U-shaped curve? In: Simopoulos AP, editor. Impacts on Nutrition and Health. World Review of Nutrition and Diet. Basel: Karger, 1991:38-71.
7.    Marmot M, Brunner E. Alcohol and cardiovascular disease: The status of the U-shaped curve. BMJ 1991;303:565-68.
8.    Poikolainen K. Epidemiologic assessment of population risks and benefits of alcohol use. Alcohol Alcoholism 1991;1(Suppl.):27-34.
9.    Jackson R, Beaglehole R. The relationship between alcohol and coronary heart disease:

Is there a protective effect? Curr Opin Lipidol 1993;4:21-26.

10. Klatsky AL. Alcohol, coronary disease, and hypertension (review). Annu Rev Med 1996;47:149-60.

11. Rimm EB, Klatsky A, Grobbee D, Stampfer MJ. Review of moderate alcohol consumption and reduced risk of coronary heart disease: Is the effect due to beer, wine, or spirits? BMJ 1996;312:731-36.

12. Rimm EB, Williams P, Fosher K, Criqui M, Stampfer MJ. A biologic basis for moderate alcohol consumption and lower coronary heart disease risk: A meta-analysis of effects on lipids and hemostatic factors. BMJ 1999;319:1523-28.

13. Rosenberg L, Slone D, Shapiro S, Kaufman DW, Miettinen OS, Stolley PD. Alcoholic beverages and myocardial infarction in young women. Am J Public Health 1981;71:82-85.

14. Yano K, Rhoads GG, Kagan A. Coffee, alcohol and risk of coronary heart disease among Japanese men living in Hawaii. N Engl J Med 1977;297:405-9.

15. Stampfer MJ, Colditz GA, Willett WC, Speizer FE, Hennekens CH. A prospective study of moderate alcohol consumption and the risk of coronary disease and stroke in women. N Engl J Med 1988;319:267-73.

16. Klatsky AL, Friedman GD, Armstrong MA. The relationship between alcoholic beverage use and other traits to blood pressure: A new Kaiser-Permanente study. Circulation 1986; 73:628-36.

17. Klatsky AL, Armstrong MA, Kipp H. Correlates of alcoholic beverage preference: Traits of persons who choose wine, liquor or beer. Br J Addict 1990;85:1279-89.

18. Rimm EB, Giovannucci E, Willett WC, et al. Alcohol and mortality. Lancet 1991;338: 1073-74.

19. Friedman LA, Kimball AW. Coronary heart disease mortality and alcohol consumption in Framingham. Am J Epidemiol 1986;124:481-89.

20. Grønbæk M, Deis A, Sorensen TIA, Becker U, Schnohr P, Jensen G. Mortality associated with moderate intakes of wine, beer, or spirits. BMJ 1995;310:1165-69.

21. Marques-Vidal P, Ducimetiere P, Evans A, et al. Alcohol consumption and myocardial infarction: A case-control study in France and Northern Ireland. Am J Epidemiol 1996; 143:1089-93.

22. Gaziano JM, Hennekens CH, Godfried SL, et al. Type of alcoholic beverage and risk of myocardial infarction. Am J Cardiol 1999;83:52-57.

23. Renaud SC, Guéguen R, Siest G, Salamon R. Wine, beer, and mortality in middle-aged men from Eastern France. Arch Intern Med 1999;159:1865-70.

24. Yuan J, Ross RK, Gao Y, et al. Follow up study of moderate alcohol intake and mortality among middle aged men in Shanghai, China. BMJ 1997;314:18-23.

25. Keil U, Chambless LE, Döring A, Filipiak B, Stieber J. The relation of alcohol intake to coronary heart disease and all-cause mortality in a beer-drinking population. Epidemiology 1997;8:150-56.

26. Fuchs CS, Stampfer MJ, Colditz GA, et al. Alcohol consumption and mortality among women. N Engl J Med 1995;332:1245-50.

27. Schnall PL, Schwartz JE, Landsbergis PA, Warren K, Pickering TG. Relation between job strain, alcohol, and ambulatory blood pressure. Hypertension 1992;19:488-94.

28. Maxwell S, Cruickshank A, Thorpe G. Red wine and antioxidant activity in serum. Lancet 1994;344:193.

29. Fitzpatrick DF, Hirschfield SL, Coffey RG. Endothelium-dependent vasorelaxing activity of wine and other grape products. Am J Physiol 1993;265:H774-H778.

30. Kluft C, Veenstra J, Schaafsma G, Pikaar NA. Regular moderate wine consumption for five weeks increases plasma activity of the plasminogen activator inhibitor-1 (PAI-1) in healthy young volunteers. Fibrinolysis 1990;4(Suppl.):69-70.

31. Renaud SC, Ruf JC. Effects of alcohol on platelet functions. Clin Chimica Acta 1996; 246:77-89.

32. Tjonneland A, Grønbæk M, Stripp C, Overvad K. Wine intake and diet in a random sample of 48763 Danish men and women. Am J Clin Nutr 1999;69:49-54.

33. Criqui M. The reduction of coronary heart disease with light to moderate alcohol consumption: Effect or artifact? Br J Addict 1990;85:854-57.

34. Criqui MH, Cowan LD, Tyroler HA, et al. Lipoproteins as mediators for the effects of alcohol consumption and cigarette smoking on cardiovascular mortality: Results from the Lipid Research Clinics Follow-up Study. Am J Epidemiol 1987;126:629-37.

35. Langer RD, Criqui MH, Reed DM. Lipoproteins and blood pressure as biological pathways for effect of moderate alcohol consumption on coronary heart disease. Circulation 1992;85:910-15.

36. Suh I, Shaten J, Cutler JA, Kuller L. Alcohol use and mortality from coronary heart disease: The role of high-density lipoprotein cholesterol. Ann Intern Med 1992;116:881-87.

37. Gaziano JM, Buring JE, Breslow JL, et al. Moderate alcohol intake, increased levels of high-density lipoprotein and its subfractions and decreased risk of myocardial infarction. N Engl J Med 1993;329:1829-34.

38. Meade TW, Chakrabarti R, Haines AP, North WR, Stirling Y. Characteristics affecting fibrinolytic activity and plasma fibrinogen concentrations. BMJ 1979;1:153-56.

39. Mikhailidis DP, Jeremy JY, Barradas A, et al. Effect of ethanol on vascular prostacyclin (prostaglan oodin $I_2$) synthesis, platelet aggregation, and platelet thromboxane release. BMJ 1983;287:1495-98.

40. Renaud SC, Beswick AD, Fehily AM, Sharp DS, Elwood PC. Alcohol and platelet aggregation: The Caerphilly prospective heart disease study. Am J Clin Nutr 1992;55:1012-17.

41. Kiechl S, Willeit J, Poewe W, et al. Insulin sensitivity and regular alcohol consumption: Large, prospective, cross sectional population study (Bruneck study). BMJ 1996;313:1040-44.

42. Vitelli LL, Folsom AR, Shahar E, et al. Association of dietary composition with fasting serum insulin level - the ARIC study. Nutr Metab Cardiovasc Dis 1996;6:194-202.

# Index

134